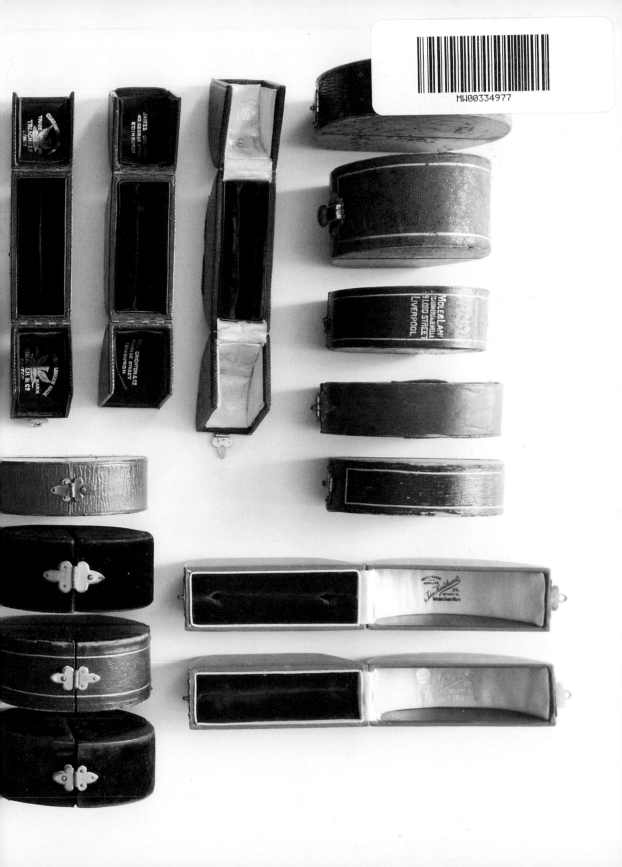

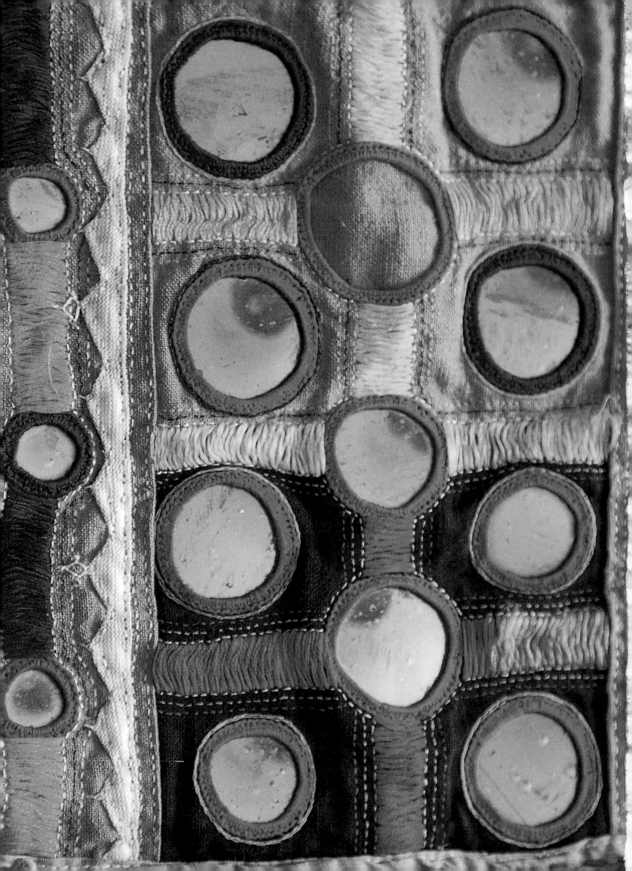

# Life in a Box

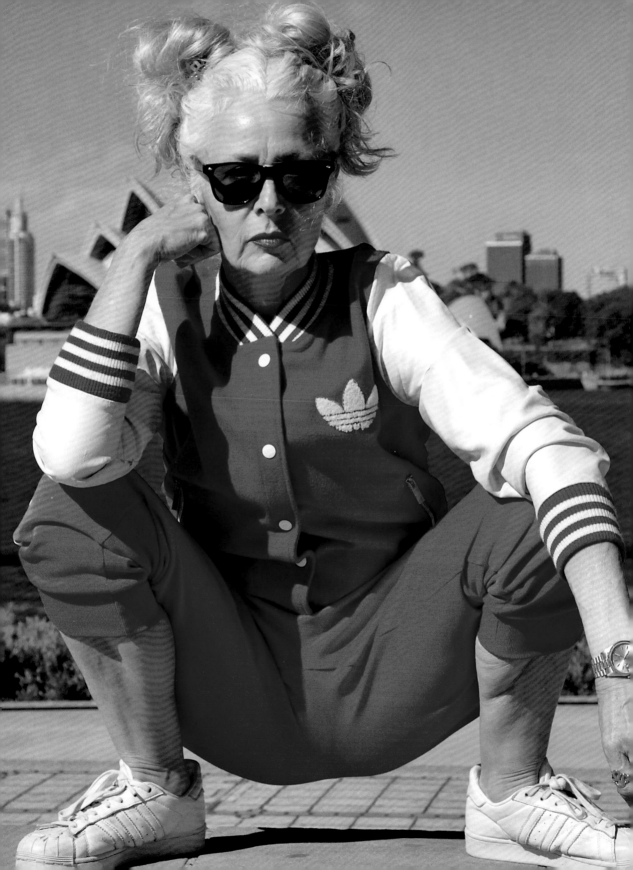

**TRAVELLER · ANTIQUES DEALER · MOTHER**
**MODEL · ICONOCLAST**

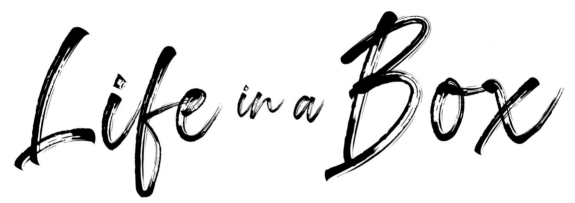

An unorthodox memoir by
## Sarah Jane Adams

PHOTOGRAPHY BY **DAVID JAMES TAYLOR**

**murdoch books**
Sydney | London

# dedication

This book is dedicated to my twin daughters, Olivia and Natasha, who aren't particularly interested in this stuff, and to Big Man, who isn't interested in stuff at all.

You three are the stuff of my world.

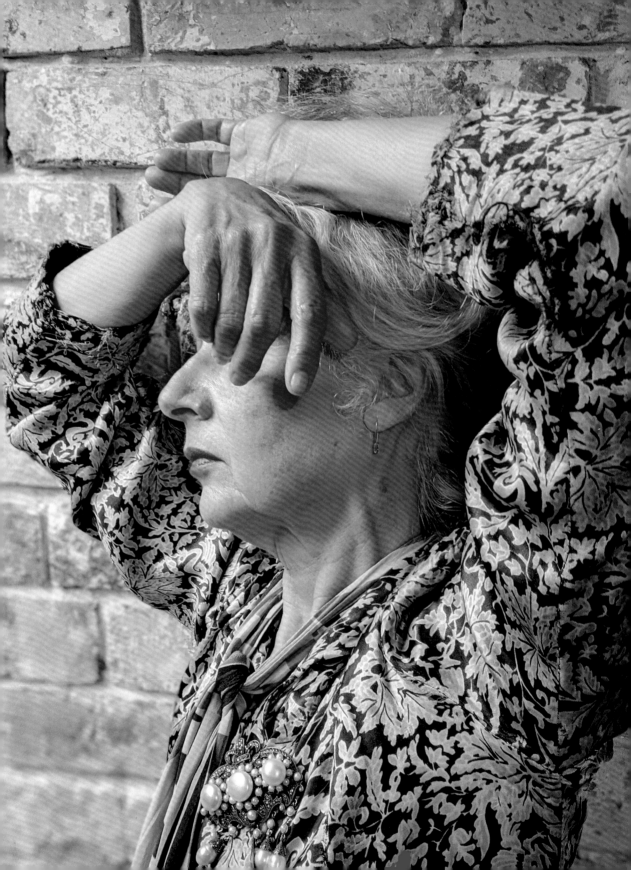

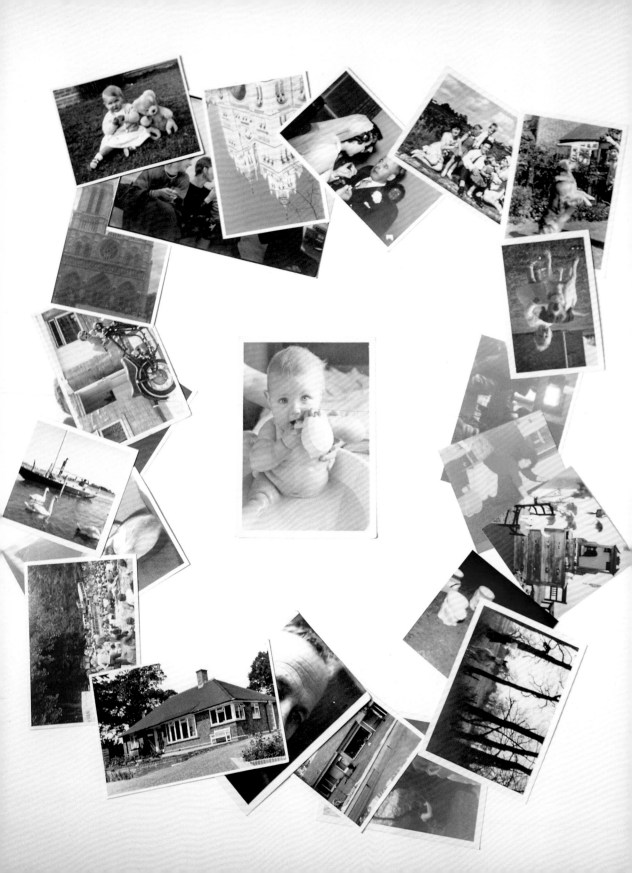

# *contents*

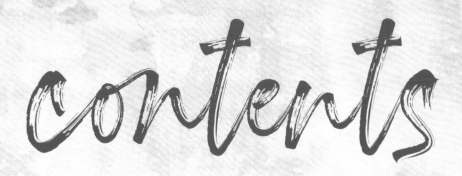

# *foreword*

My first introduction to Sarah Jane Adams was through an Instagram photo of her dressed in a red and white Adidas sports jacket and matching head scarf, her arms folded, exposing a gold Rolex watch and henna tattoos along her hands. She gazed directly at the camera with a strength and nonchalance that aligned perfectly with what I would come to know as one of her most common statements: "I can't be bothered." She was (and is) the coolest woman I had ever seen.

Sarah hated having her picture taken. She might wonder, what was the point? The story goes that on this particular day someone had made a 'smart-ass' comment about the way she was dressed. In reaction, Sarah asked her husband, DT (Big Man), to take a photo of her in the jacket, which her daughter then put on Sarah's antique jewellery Instagram page with the hashtags #advancedstyle #mymumiscoolerthanme.

I was just about to leave Sydney, travelling for a tour for the release of my documentary film, *Advanced Style*, when this powerful image popped up on my Instagram feed. I quickly commented, asking where it was taken and, when I read Sydney in the reply, I asked if I could meet and take a photo of Sarah on my way to the airport and back to the US the next day.

Her daughter arranged for us to meet, with Sarah not having a clue of what was going on, who I was and why I would want her photograph. She reluctantly allowed me to take a few snaps, which I later posted online. These images instantly went viral – not because of the clothes Sarah wore, but the attitude with which she wore them.

A single mother, jewellery designer, fighter and storyteller, Sarah has been defying people's expectations ever since she was a little girl. Everything she does is an act of rebellion against the conventional, the bullshit, the mundane and the inauthentic. She is on a constant quest for authenticity, fuelled by an intense curiosity and a need to share the mysteries of life through subtle cues and messages. Her objects, clothing and jewellery serve as a diary and road map of her life's journey and lessons. They also serve to protect her from revealing too much of her inherent hypersensitivity, empathy and vulnerability. The lucky ones who push past these protective layers will quickly discover her incredible generosity of spirit, a fierce loyalty and an understanding that it's almost impossible for Sarah Jane Adams to be anything other than who she is, to do anything other than what she feels. I am grateful to be one of these lucky few.

*Ari Seth Cohen*

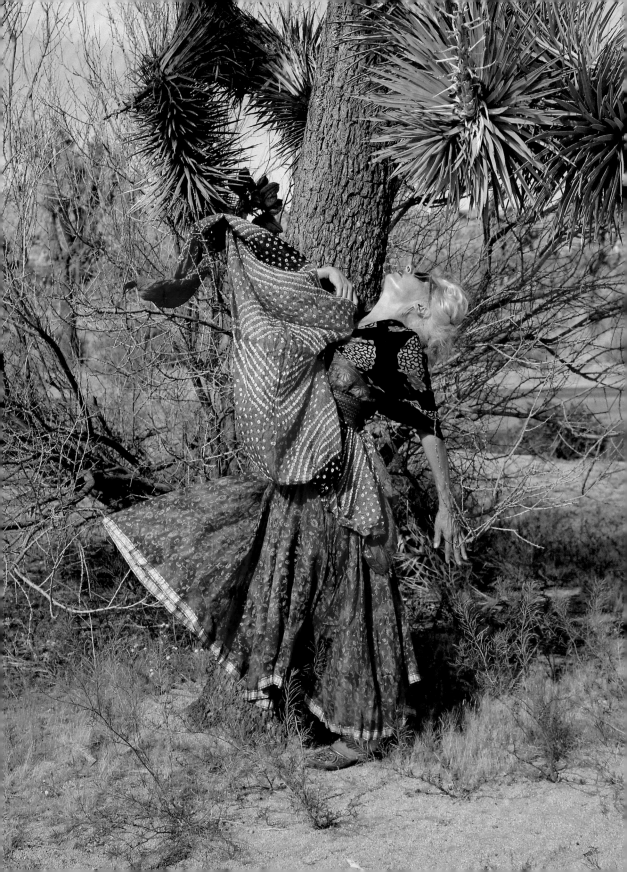

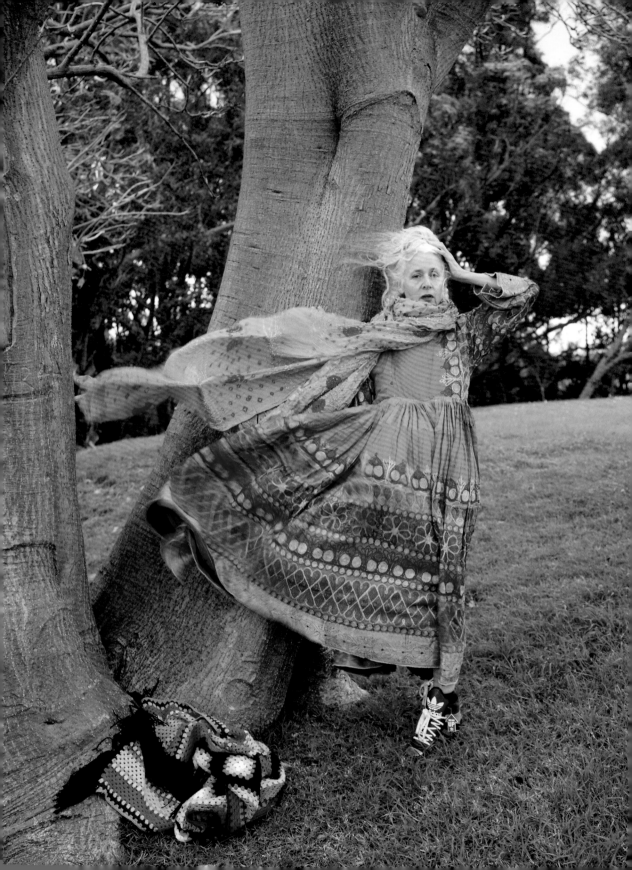

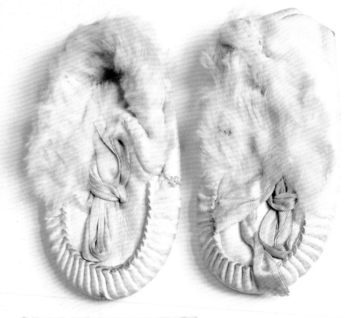
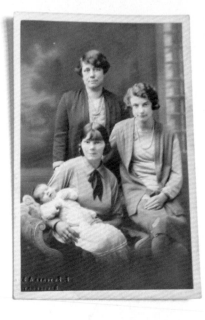
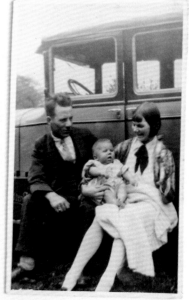
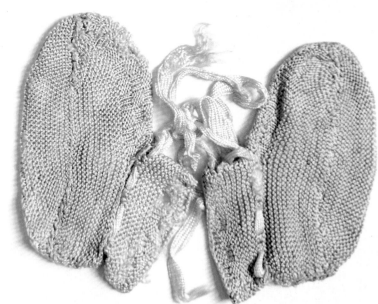

LOT **6**

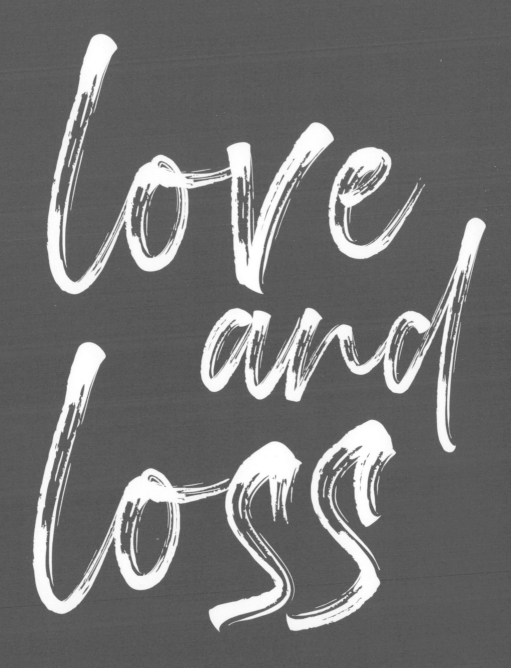

# CHAPTER 1

## LOT 1

### TWO COTTON DRESSES, c1992 (ONE PICTURED), TWO PHOTOGRAPHS, c1900, AND ONE PHOTOGRAPH, 1992

$20–$30

Twins, twins, twins. Three generations of twins in one family. The photographs taken in the late 1800s show my paternal grandfather and his twin sister with their nanny and an older sibling. The colour photograph is of my twin daughters in their sailor dresses.

The Victorian children are all dressed in sailor suits, a cute version of the uniforms worn by the British Royal Navy, which, at that time, was kept very busy expanding the British Empire. Patriotism was reflected in all areas of life, fashion being one of them. Nostalgia, rather than patriotism, was my reason for dressing my daughters this way.

I was also born a twin. Twindom does not skip a generation.

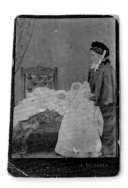
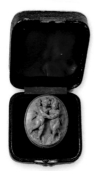

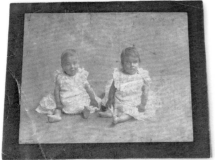

## LOT 2

### LAVA CAMEO BROOCH OF TWO CHERUBS IN A BRASS FRAME, BOXED, c1850

$300–$350

The Victorian-era brooch is hand-carved and depicts two 'putti' – winged cherubs holding bows and arrows. It would most likely have been carved in Italy, and the cherubs represent love and loss. I have a fascination with 'twin' jewellery, as twins are common in my family: the boy twin in the photographs is my paternal grandfather; I was the firstborn of twins; and I am also the mother of Gemini twin girls, now all grown up.

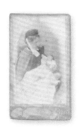
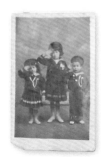
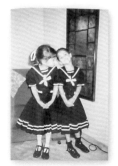

Nostalgia, rather than patriotism, was my reason for dressing my daughters this way.

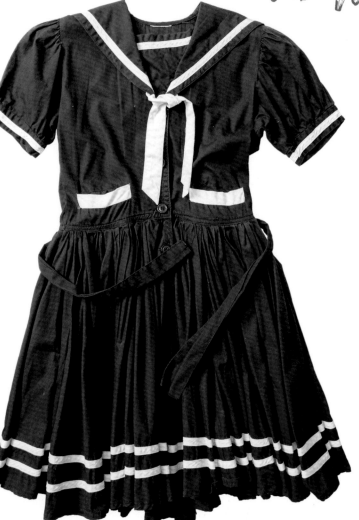

LOT **1**

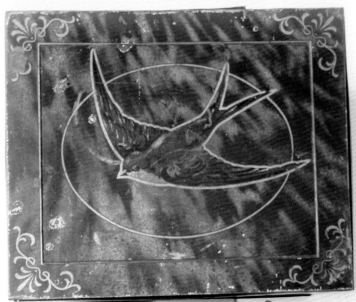

Nanny Win's 'Life in a Box'

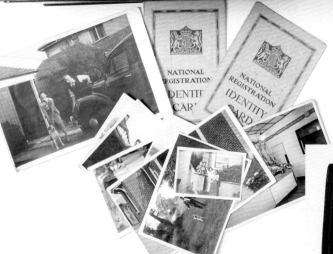

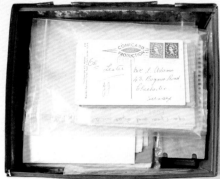

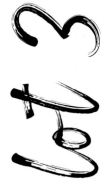

Lot 3

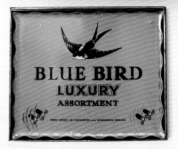

BLUE BIRD
LUXURY
ASSORTMENT

## LOT **3**

### BLUE BIRD 'LUXURY ASSORTMENT' BISCUIT TIN (HINGE BROKEN), CONTAINING PHOTOGRAPHS AND VARIOUS CORRESPONDENCE, c1910

$30–$40

This is my paternal grandmother, Nanny Win's, 'Life in a Box'. When I was little, we would secretly open it together and she would share her memories, her deepest thoughts, wishes, regrets and tales of her life and times. It was this tin full of memories that gave me the title for this book and taught me to recognise, extract and condense the meaningful from the mundane.

## LOT **4**

### HANDWRITTEN LETTER, DATED 27 APRIL 1904

$5–$10

A letter from the suitor of my grandmother's biological mother to her father: *"You scoundrel you have ruined my affianced wife, and my life, and may God's curse rest upon you for this evil done. Tis well such a distance separates us for I could shoot you like a dog. Look to yourself, if we ever meet again, one of us will suffer."*

Nanny Win was the result of a liaison between her father, a businessman in Portsmouth, and one of his housemaids. His wife had born him no children and when the maid's pregnancy was discovered the two women were sent away together. The wife returned home with the baby – my grandmother – who, sadly, never saw her biological mother again.

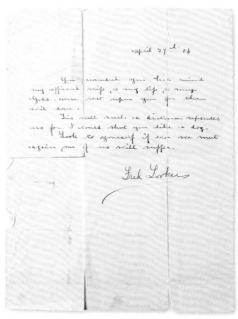

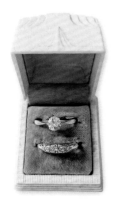

## LOT 5

### TWO DIAMOND RINGS IN PRESENTATION BOX, c1930

$350–$450

These were my grandmother's engagement and eternity rings. I remember when I was young, the rings spent much of their time on the kitchen windowsill or hidden in the airing cupboard, as my grandmother was always doing things. When she wasn't busy cleaning, cooking or looking after me, she was outdoors with nature, gardening or taking long walks with the dog. I sensed that this was when she was her most contented self. These two items were her most valuable and I wonder, for how much of her life were they also the most precious?

## LOT 6

### TWO PAIRS OF BABY'S BOOTIES AND
### TWO PHOTOGRAPHS, c1930 (SHOWN ON PAGE 12)

$30–$40

From my grandmother's 'Life in a Box' (Lot 3), one pair made of white rabbit skin with pale blue ribbon, the other being pale blue knitted cotton. My grandmother is seen holding my father as a baby in both photographs.

## LOT 7

### FOUR LOCKS OF HAIR WRAPPED IN PAPER
### AND TWO PHOTOGRAPHS, c1930

$5–$10

The hair is that of my father when he was a baby, cut in the 1930s and saved in folded paper with my grandmother's handwriting indicating his age at the time of the haircut. The photos show my father as a toddler. These items were kept in my grandmother's 'Life in a Box', which I loved to look through with her. Her stories made me feel connected in ways that I couldn't yet understand, and were stronger than the connections I felt in this life.

# These items were kept in my grandmother's 'Life in a Box'

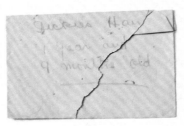

Dickie boy's hair

Dickies Hair 1 year old 9 months old

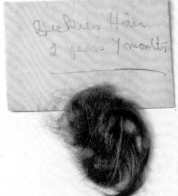

Dickies Hair 2 years 7 months

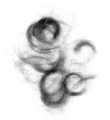

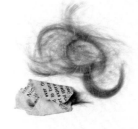

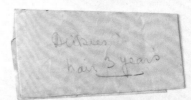

Dickies hair 5 years

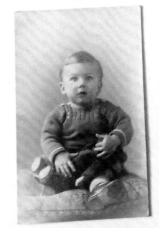

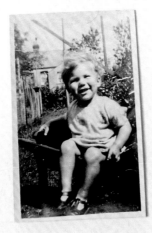

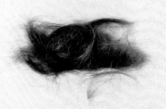

## CHICKEN WISHBONE MADE INTO THE FIGURE OF A SOLDIER, c1940

$20–$30

This handmade figure was made at Shippam's, an English food company founded in 1750 by Shipston Shippam of Chichester. Shippam's was famous for its meat and fish pastes, which were produced in its factory in East Street. The stench that emanated from that part of town still lingers in my upper nostrils, and I recall being told it was the smell of horses' hooves being boiled to make the jelly for the pastes.

My mother had two older half-brothers. My maternal grandmother had been married to a member of the Shippam family, the father of these two boys. Tragically, along with so many others, he lost his life in World War I and my grandmother was widowed with two small boys to raise. Mr Shippam senior, realising how difficult life as a single mother would be, purchased a property for my grandmother and here she opened the first fish and chip shop in Chichester. It was in the fish and chip shop that she subsequently met my mother's father.

So, I have a fragile connection to the Shippam family and this is how I know about the wishbone characters, the forerunners of the plastic toys given away today by food companies. I assume that not many of these little lucky wishbone people have stood the test of time, due to their fragility, low value and the lack of information about them. However, if you're a Shippam, this one-off little guy is a priceless part of your family history.

*lucky wishbone*

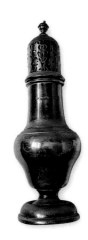

## LOT **9**

### EDWARDIAN SUGAR SHAKER (BENT AT BASE), HALLMARKED STERLING SILVER (HMSS), SB&S LTD, CHESTER, 1936

$250–$300

This is one of a few family heirlooms – a silver sugar shaker, which doesn't stand up straight, and from whom I can't remember. I don't use sugar.

## LOT **10**

### SET OF SIX FOLEY CHINA TEA CUPS AND SAUCERS, c1940

$80–$100 (WITHDRAWN)

These cups and saucers came from the estate of my maternal grandmother. They remain unused and unpacked, in a cardboard box with a few other family items. Although they are small and of little value, I am not quite yet ready to get rid of them.

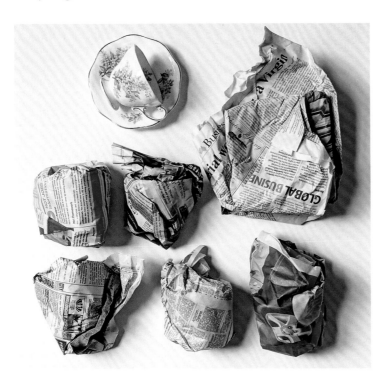

## LOT 11

### TWO HANDWRITTEN LETTERS CONCERNING THE ADOPTION OF A CHILD, DATED 1904 AND 1905

$5–$10

The child about whom the letters are written, referred to as "It", is my paternal grandmother, Nanny Win. (See Lot 4 for details of her parentage.) She showed me these letters and, even though I was a very young child, I felt the trauma she suffered surrounding her start in life and her sense of identity. Now, as an adult, I recognise the courage shown by her adopted mother, a woman who had the moral strength and mental fortitude to publicly adopt the illegitimate child of another woman fathered by her husband. I deeply hope that my grandmother came to understand how much she was wanted and loved.

## LOT 12

### PHOTOGRAPH WITH INSCRIPTION ON REVERSE "MY MOTHER AND STEPSISTER, SOUTH AFRICA", c1920

NCV (NO COMMERCIAL VALUE, WITHDRAWN)

This is the only photograph in existence of the mother and stepsister my grandmother never knew (see Lot 11). The older woman is my biological great-grandmother, and I sense a connection. This photograph was my grandmother's secret, which she guiltily, emotionally and stoically shared with me. It is in safe hands now.

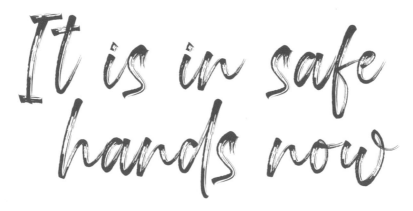

*It is in safe hands now*

90, Bargates,
Christchurch,
Hants,

30 MAY 1905 190

Dear Miss Rogers

Enclosed please find the
Birth Certificate you asked
me to obtain for you. You will
see that the child will now be
called by the name given in
Col 10 instead of that given
in Col. 2.

Yours faithfully
Ernest G. Marshall

Miss Rogers
Sharpnels,
Bittern Park
SOUTHAMPTON.

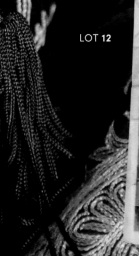

LOT 12

36 Porchester Road.
Woolston
Sept 15th /04

My dear Mrs Mumford.

In answer to your
letter of this morning. We
are quite willing for you
to adopt the little child,
for we feel sure you will
act as a Mother towards
it. and we cannot suf-
ficiently thank you
for your kind and noble
offer. Will you kindly
let me know your plans
and when you would

LOT 11

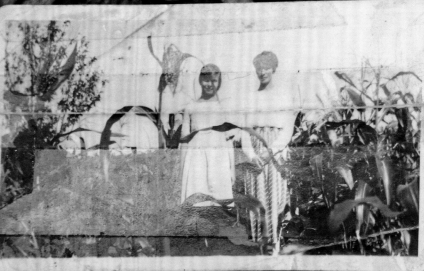

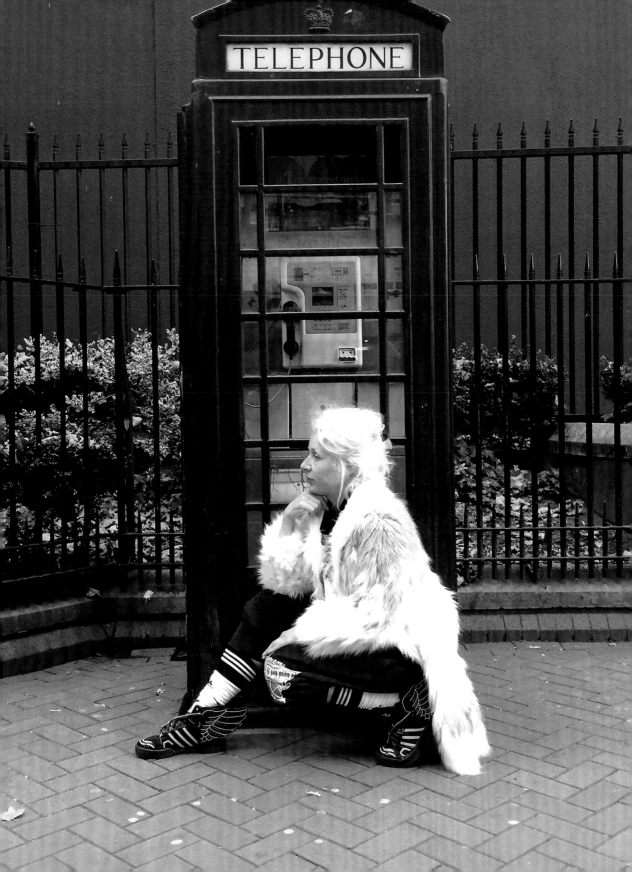

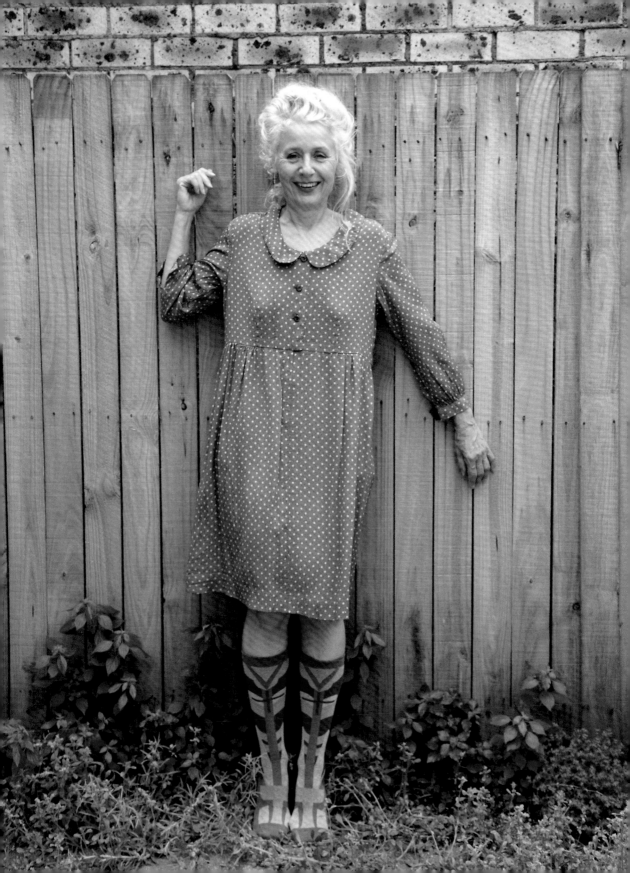

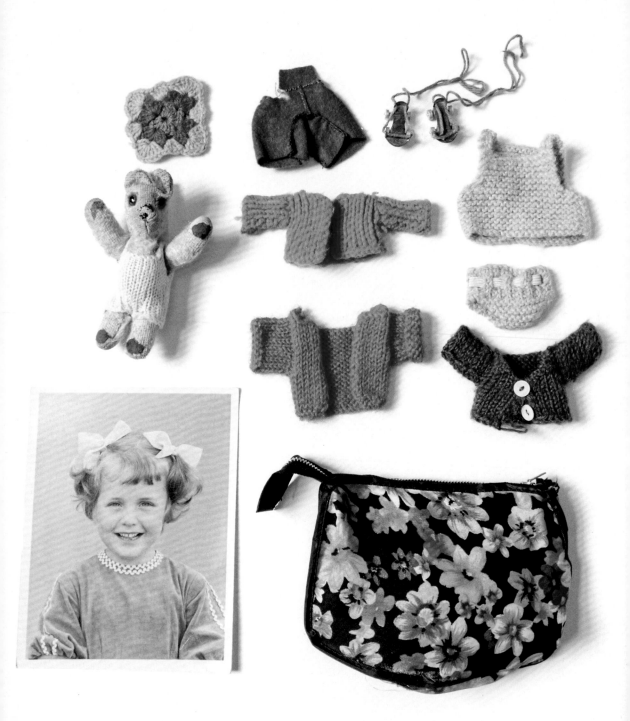

LOT **21**

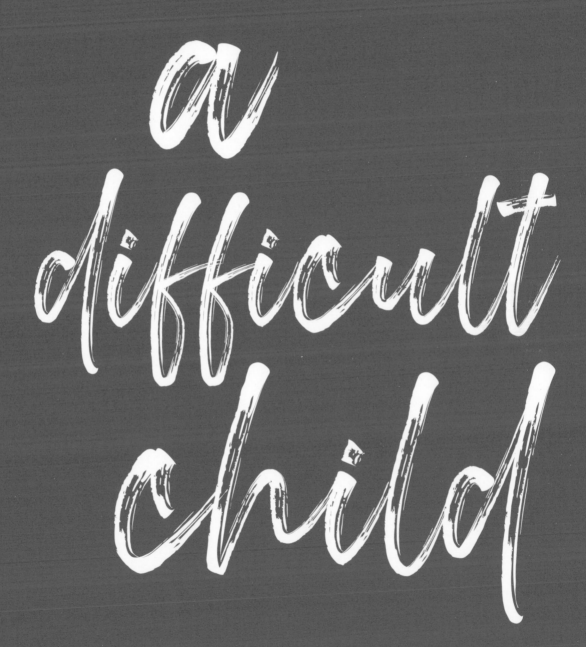

a difficult child

## CHILD'S SILVER BRACELET (DAMAGED), WITH PHOTOGRAPHS AND OTHER EPHEMERA

NCV (WITHDRAWN)

I entered the world in this body on 16 April 1955. My mother, who was expecting twins, had a difficult pregnancy, as she was suffering from pre-eclampsia, thereby needing to spend much of her time in hospital on bed rest. I was the first-born baby. My birth was 'difficult' (a word used to describe me from that day forth). Mother needed much medication to deliver me; I was led to believe from a very young age that this medication took the life force from my sister, who was stillborn two days after me.

The small announcement in the *Chichester Observer* tells nothing of the trauma that must have been endured by all concerned at the time of birth. Apparently, my father passed out in the delivery room and had to be sent home. I have never spoken in detail about my birth, only ever as a matter of fact. These, I believe, are the facts.

The accompanying numbered photographs show my mother in happier times as the St Pancras beauty queen (1), not looking so happy on the day her pregnancy was announced (2), and in hospital soon after my birth (3). Nurse Nisbett (4) was apparently the first person to hold the newly delivered baby. The baptism was held four weeks later in Donnington Parish Church (5). Later in life, being 'difficult', I chose not to attend confirmation classes at school.

*My birth was 'difficult' (a word used to describe me from that day forth).*

**1.**

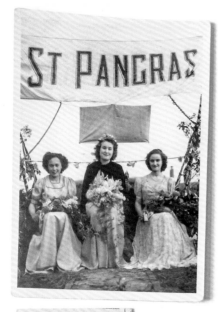

St PANCRAS

**2.**

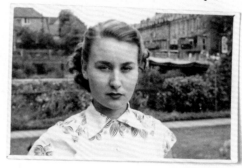

**4.**

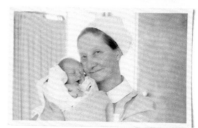

**3.**

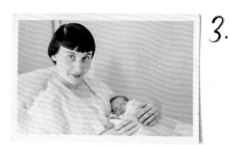

BIRTHS, MARRIAGES
AND DEATHS

BIRTHS

ADAMS—To Richard and Dorothy (nee Welch), the gift of a daughter on April 16, at Zachary Merton Maternity Hospital Sarah Jane. 17.
STRONG — On April 23rd, at Rustington, to Ivy (nee Galloway) and Robert, a daughter (Lindsay Ann). 17.

ENGAGEMENTS

BUDD—HARFIELD — The engagement is announced between P.O. Brian F. Budd, E.R.A., elder son of Mr. and Mrs. P. W. H. Budd, of The Kennels, Goodwood, and Marjorie, elder daughter of Mr. and Mrs. W. Harfield, of Purbrook, Hants. 62.
BURLINSON — KNIGHT — The engagement is announced between David Maurice Theodore, son of Mr. and Mrs. J. M. Burlinson, of 22, Glenwood Grove, London, N.W.9, and Jennifer, daughter of Mr. and Mrs. P. H. Knight of Mr. and Mrs. ...

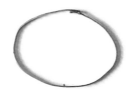

**5.**

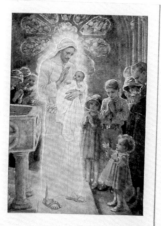

Behold, what manner of love the Father hath bestowed upon us that we should be called children of God.

SARAH JANE

was baptised

at St. George's DUNNINGTON PARISH CHURCH

on SUNDAY, MAY 15th 1955

by R. Humphry McKennight Vicar

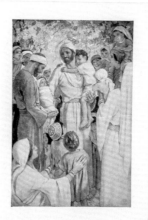

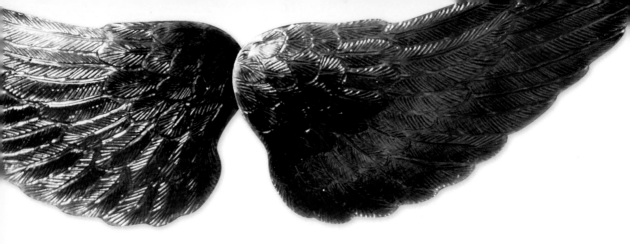

## LOT 14

### MASSIVE 'WING' BELT BUCKLE IN FITTED BOX, MEASURING 10 INCHES (25CM), SILVER WITH IRIDESCENT PURPLE ENAMEL, c1900

$800–$900

Wings represent the transcendence of the soul to a higher state; that is, a release from the human condition, freedom to leave earthly things behind and to ascend to Paradise. These wings evoke thoughts of my deceased twin sister. Although separated from her at birth, she remains with me, protecting me with a love that gives me the strength of our two forces combined. From a very young age I have felt her beside me. Later, at those times when I felt desperately alone, I acknowledged that I had experienced a very special love and the words of Alfred Lord Tennyson would soothe my soul: *"Tis better to have loved and lost/Than never to have loved at all."* (*In Memoriam*, 1850)

The buckle, which gives no hint of where and by whom it was made, was a gift from my dear friend, Kirsten Albrecht.

## LOT 15

### COLLECTION OF 'CONGRATULATIONS ON YOUR NEW BABY' CARDS, APRIL 1955

$20–$30

These cards were sent to my parents on the birth of their new baby daughter. Nowhere is there mention of my stillborn twin, other than a line: "So pleased to hear the good news, glad you've put 'Jane' in." Presumably, that is why I was given a double-barrelled Christian name, with which, by the way, I was never comfortable.

## LOT 16
## PAIR OF COSTUME CLIP-ON HOOP EARRINGS
## AND THREE PHOTOGRAPHS, MID-1950s

$10–$20

The silver-coloured hoop earrings belonged to my mother. She can be seen wearing them in the three photos of us together. My mother never pierced her ears (my father, a squeamish man, found the idea "gruesome") and, although I somehow acquired these earrings in my early teens, I've never worn them. Hoops are not my thing.

LOT **15**

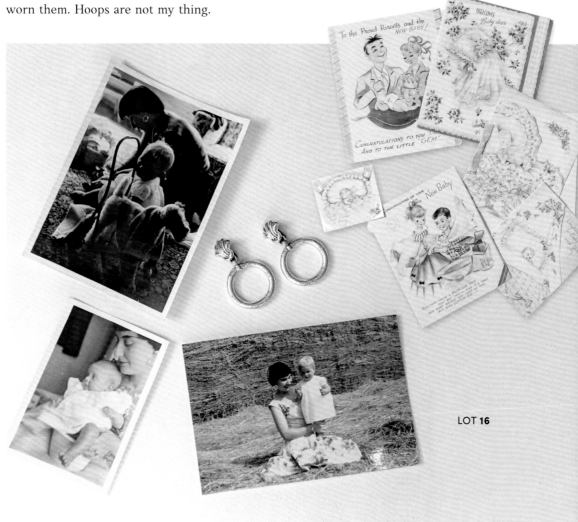

LOT **16**

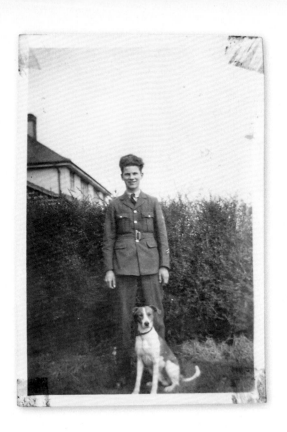

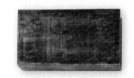

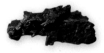

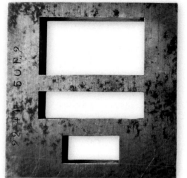

*The piece of shrapnel was my father's lucky charm.*

LOT **17**

**METALWORK APPRENTICE PIECE,
A PIECE OF SHRAPNEL, AND PHOTOGRAPH, c1945**

$20–$30

The photograph shows my father with the family dog, Sandy, taken shortly after he joined the Royal Air Force as World War II was coming to an end.

His apprentice engineer piece consists of two pieces of iron, the smaller rectangle fitting perfectly in three directions into the larger, square frame. This is the precision work that my father made as part of his studies to become an aircraft engineer.

The piece of shrapnel was my father's lucky charm. Although I'm not sure of the exact story, I'm told it saved his life by jamming into a moving aircraft engine, thereby preventing him from serious injury. When my father became a pilot after the war had come to an end, he kept this fragment of twisted metal with him on every sortie, every trip – his *memento mori* amulet.

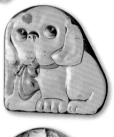

## LOT 18

### TIN BOX DECORATED WITH A DOG, J LYONS & CO LTD, CADBY HALL, LONDON W14, c1940, CONTAINING FRAGMENTS OF A 'LARRY THE LAMB' TOY, c1955

$10–$20

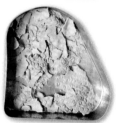

Larry the Lamb was my earliest companion. As a baby, I listened to his adventures on a BBC radio program called *Children's Hour*. Larry was a soft rubber squeeze toy that accompanied me everywhere – my initials were written onto the sole of his foot when we were packed off together to boarding school.

Many years passed. Larry was put into hibernation whilst I journeyed through secondary school, university, travel, marriage, divorce, adulthood. When the day came for me to remove my stuff from the hot roof space of my parents' house, I rediscovered Larry, fragmented in a box, yet still whole somewhere in my very distant memory.

## LOT 19

### FOUR ITEMS OF JEWELLERY, INCLUDING A RARE TASMANIAN ABORIGINAL SHELL NECKLACE, c1820, AND ONE PHOTOGRAPH, 1953

$500–$600

The photograph of my grandmothers was taken at my parents' wedding at Donnington Church in Chichester. All the items were given to me by these ladies when I was little. I remember as a very young child being completely in awe of the Tasmanian maireener shells – their incredible iridescence and natural colour were unlike anything I had ever seen before and held the utmost fascination for me. The carved-bone edelweiss brooch was one of my paternal grandmother's favourites, and I would fiddle with it when it was pinned onto her cardi. I remember being so excited the day she removed it and pinned it onto mine.

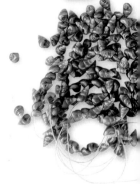

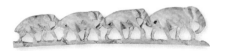

**#20**

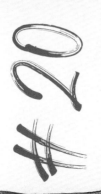

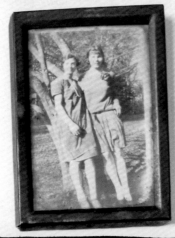

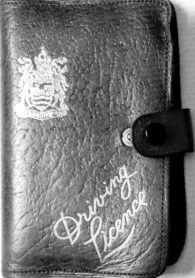

*Driving Licence*

*Autographs*

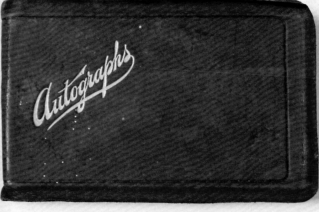

4s

*To Winnie from Mother Christmas Dec 22, 1914*

The Book of
# Common Prayer,

And Administration of the Sacraments, and other Rites and Ceremonies of the Church, according to the Use of

## The Church of England;

together with the

## Psalter or Psalms of David,

Pointed as they are to be sung or said in Churches:
and the Form and Manner of Making,
Ordaining, and Consecrating of
Bishops, Priests, and
Deacons.

London:

PRINTED BY EYRE AND SPOTTISWOODE, LTD.,
Printers to the King's most Excellent Majesty,
FOR THE
SOCIETY FOR PROMOTING CHRISTIAN KNOWLEDGE,
SOLD AT THE SOCIETY'S DEPOSITORY, NORTHUMBERLAND AVENUE,
CHARING CROSS, LONDON, W.C.

Ruby 32mo.

## LOT 20

## AUTOGRAPH BOOK, *THE BOOK OF COMMON PRAYER*, DRIVING LICENCE, NEWSPAPER CLIPPING, AND PHOTOGRAPH, c1930

$60–$80

These items all belonged to my favourite grandmother, Winifred Adams, seen here in a photograph along with her obituary, clipped from the newspaper.

Before social media, our 'followers' expressed their 'likes' and 'comments' in a very different way – the autograph book. At the turn of the 20th century, the autograph book was a tangible, very personal and often highly sentimental way of collecting memories, messages and thoughts from loved ones, family members and folk who shared a moment in one's life.

As a small child, I spent many an afternoon with Nanny Win, going through her own autograph books, as she reminisced about people and recalled their stories. The handwritten experiences they'd shared were captured for all time on a page in this soft, shabby, leather-bound book; a microcosm of days together and times gone by. I sensed the comfort my grandmother drew from them as she tenderly caressed those pages, the messages contained in them evoking thoughts that brought tears and a faraway look to her eyes. I wondered if I would ever understand this world of grown-ups and their mysteries.

## LOT 21

## SMALL TEDDY BEAR WITH CLOTHES IN A SATIN BAG, AND PHOTOGRAPH c1960 (SHOWN ON PAGE 26)

$40–$60

I spent a lot of time at my grandparents' house in Chichester. There was a big barn at the bottom of the garden, where boxes of different-sized brown paper bags were stored, which my grandfather delivered to the small shops in the area. I remember climbing and jumping on these piles of boxes, and occasionally I went with my Grandpa on his rounds.

One day I spotted this tiny teddy, who became known as Tessie Bear, tucked behind the rear-view mirror of his delivery van. By the end of the journey, she had become mine. My mother and grandmother were tasked with the job of dressing Tessie Bear.

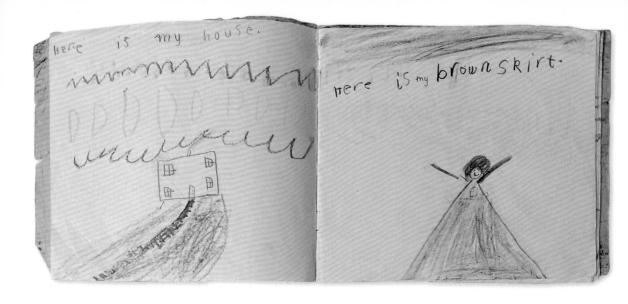

## LOT **22**

### CHILD'S DRAWING BOOK WITH SKETCHES,
### AND PHOTOGRAPH, c1960

$5–$10

'My Story Book by Sarah Jane Adams' is my primary-school drawing book.
The page is opened at the picture 'Here is my brown skirt', an item of
clothing that clearly made a big impression. In the photograph, Tessie Bear
(Lot 21) is in my right hand, dressed in her red cardi (my, and her,
favourite colour).

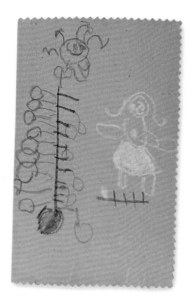

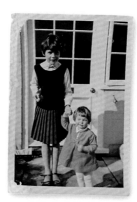

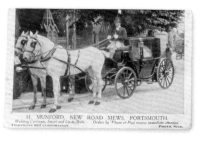

## LOT 23
## VICTORIAN SILVER HORSESHOE BROOCH, TWO SEPIA PHOTOGRAPHS, c1910, AND AUTOGRAPH BOOK WITH DRAWING, c1966

$50–$100

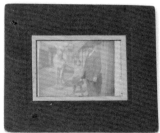

The silver horseshoe brooch belonged to my grandmother, Nanny Win, seen right as a little girl holding the reins to the big grey horse. The photo above shows horses pulling a carriage for the family business. As a young girl, if the function was a happy one, such as a wedding, she would be dressed in all her finery and allowed to drive the horses that pulled the carriage.

In medieval times, the horseshoe represented protection from evil. The iron from which the shoe was forged could withstand fire, so when women who were thought to be witches were subsequently burnt at the stake, a horseshoe was placed on the witch's grave to prevent her resurrection.

In Victorian jewellery, the horseshoe was a common motif, symbolising protection and good fortune. It had long been a commonly held belief that if a horseshoe was placed upside-down, one's luck would 'run out'. This horseshoe, which was once my grandmother's, provides me with many memories that won't be lost, regardless of which way up it's hung!

Nanny Win was an avid animal-rights activist. Every year at the time of the Grand National – a punishing steeplechase – she would campaign for the welfare of the horses. On the day of the race she would be distraught, as injury and subsequent euthanasia were common occurrences.

The drawing in her autograph book was done by me, aged 11.

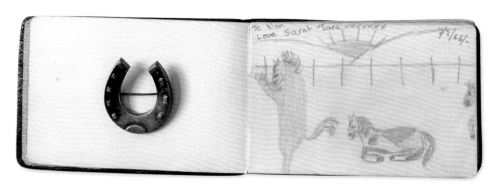

LOT **24**

## MINIATURE REPLICA OF THE *SUNDAY TELEGRAPH,* 4 FEBRUARY 1962

$25–$40

This miniature newspaper measures 4 inches by 5½ inches (10cm by 14cm). It was the first thing I ever really wanted to own (after Tessie Bear) – a gift that came with my grandfather's *Sunday Telegraph* – and I was entranced by its size, cuteness and seriousness. It was a tantalising symbol of a grown-up world, a world in which I had no part. Mine was one where children should be seen and not heard. I hoped that through osmosis I might find out what secrets lay in its pages, and possibly get a glimpse into that other world.

LOT **25**

## TWO HOLY BIBLES AND TWO COMMON PRAYER BOOKS, WITH INSCRIPTIONS (WORN)

$10–$20

Inscriptions read: 'To Sarah Jane from Nannie Win and Grandpa Adams, Christmas 1960', and 'To Sarah Jane from Mummy and Daddy, Christmas 1966'. Exciting Christmas reading for a five-year-old and an 11-year-old.

LOT **26**

## LADY'S WRISTWATCH, c1950, COPPER BANGLE AND TWO BUTTERFLY TRINKETS, WITH TWO PHOTOGRAPHS, c1960 AND c1975

$10–$20

The photos show Nanny Win with two of her beloved dogs, Honey Bee and Beauty. She was practical and resourceful, and the plain wristwatch and copper bracelet, which "kept the arthritis at bay", were her staple accessories. She was a nature lover who would go for long rambles across the fields, walking home beside a row of poplar trees like those in a series by Claude Monet. The day our photo was taken, I had to stand with my legs tightly crossed as I was desperate to do a pee! We're both wearing handknits made by Nanny Win – earthy colours were, and still are, amongst my favourites.

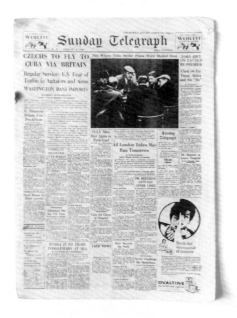

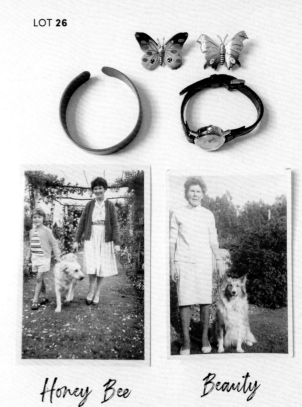

*Honey Bee*    *Beauty*

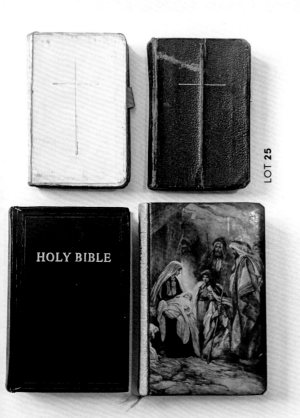

To Nan.

SARAH JANE

A Pup from the
"RUNNING
FOXES"

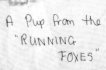

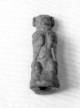

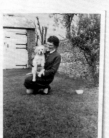

## LOT 27

### VICTORIAN HANDMADE TERRACOTTA DOG WHISTLE, c1900, DRAWING, c1967, AND PHOTOGRAPH, c1965

$50–$80

I did this drawing for Nanny Win. The photograph shows her with her beloved golden retriever, Honey Bee, in the back garden in Chichester.

## LOT 28

### MOKO JUNIOR 'MUFFIN THE MULE' FINGER PUPPET, c1950, AND MINIATURE 'MUFFIN' TOY, c1960

$150–$200

I'm sure that many people of my generation will remember Annette Mills (in monochrome on the television) cheerfully greeting us with "Hello everyone, have you seen Muffin?" followed by her singing, "We want Muffin, Muffin the Mule, dear old Muffin, playing the fool," as Muffin trotted along the top of the piano to whisper in her ear.

Although as a child I didn't have any Muffin toys, I couldn't resist this trip down memory lane when, many years later, I found him in a flea market. The puppet with four original strings with finger rings attached was produced in the 1950s by Lesney Products & Co Ltd for Moko, before it was bought out by Matchbox.

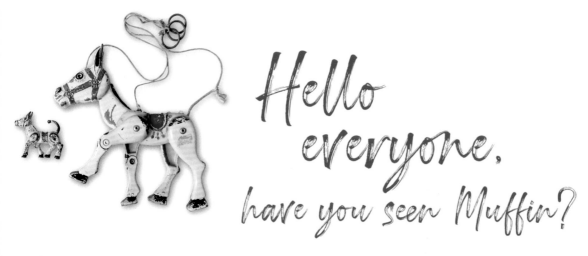

*Hello everyone, have you seen Muffin?*

## LOT 29
### 9CT GOLD BRACELET WITH PADLOCK CLASP, SET WITH THREE CABOCHON GARNETS, IN BOX, c1880
$550–$650

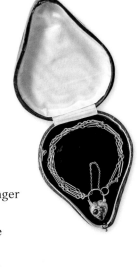

This bracelet came from my mother's side of the family. I loved the fat little padlock, which somehow warmed my heart. The chain, however, never really *felt* right. My mother told me that it had been part of a longer chain, which had been cut into short sections and distributed amongst the children. Later, as an antiques dealer, I learnt that this is one of the reasons that a good, full-length guard chain is so scarce.

Throughout history, jewellery has been modified, altered and broken into component bits and pieces to be shared amongst loved ones. Generally, each time this happens, the component parts are worth less in monetary value than if they remained in their original form. So, my attachment to this bracelet perfectly illustrates the sentimental, rather than financial, value of an item of jewellery.

## LOT 30
### RED, WHITE AND BLUE PROPELLING PENCIL WITH DICE, c1940
$5–$10

This chubby little pencil was given to me by my Great Aunt Eileen, my grandfather's twin sister. Aunt Eileen lived alone in an apartment near the English Channel and, on occasion I would accompany Nanny Win to visit her.

Aunty Eileen's home was exotic, filled with intriguing paraphernalia the likes of which I had never seen before. I remember being in awe (almost frightened by) but attracted to this flamboyant woman, whom my grandmother told me had been an actress and a model. The little pencil was in her handbag and I was fascinated by it; not just by the colours – patriotic red, white and blue – but because it felt so good. It was comfortable, sitting in my small hand, my finger hooked through the short chain from which the dice hung. It came home with me and became one of my special treasures, alien, yet familiar.

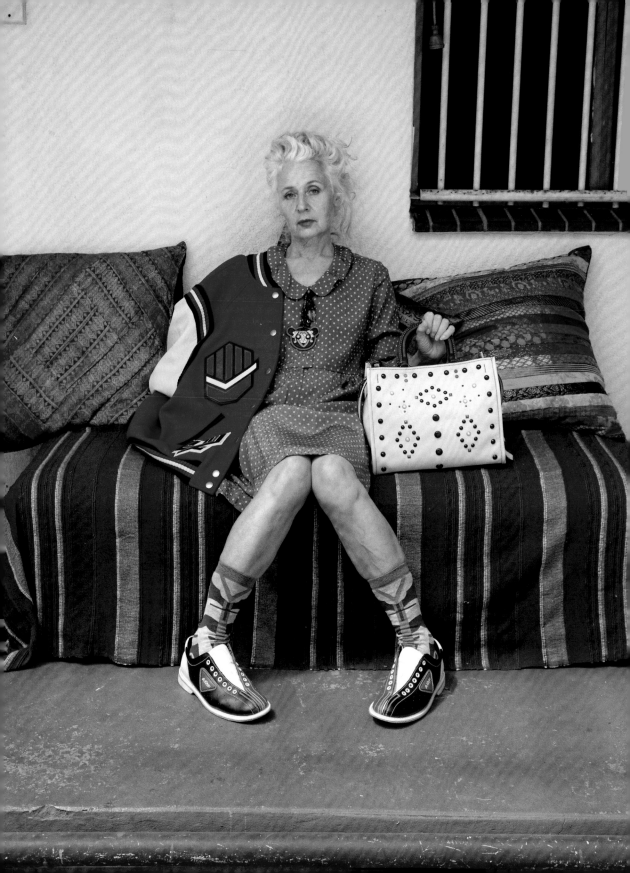

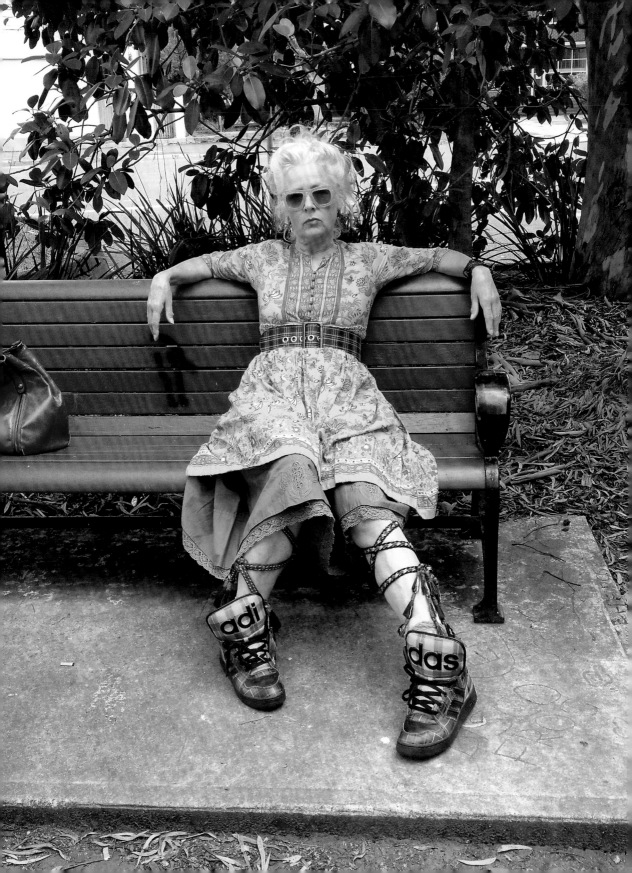

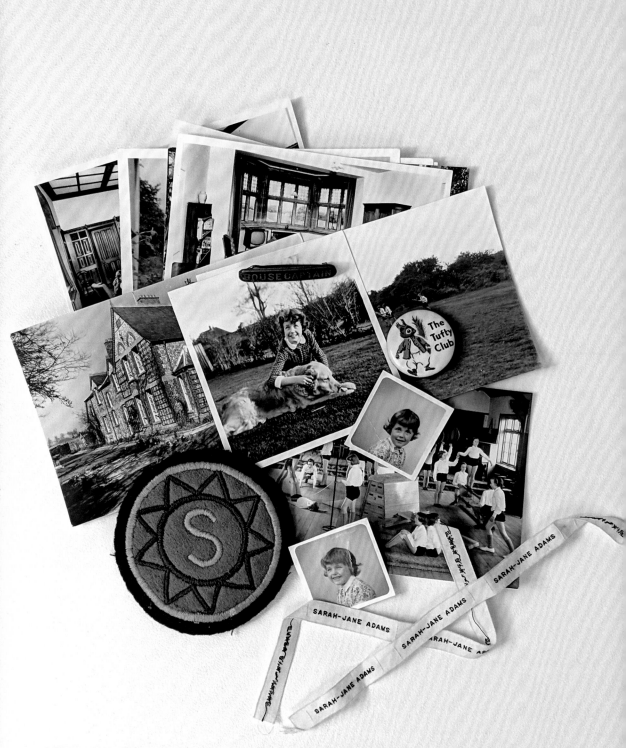

# my secret identity

## SELECTION OF BLACK-AND-WHITE PHOTOGRAPHS, EMBROIDERED 'S' BADGE, NAME TAGS, ENAMEL 'HOUSE CAPTAIN' BADGE AND 'THE TUFTY CLUB' PIN, c1960

$15–$20

The small, square photographs were taken the day I was kitted out in my new school uniform. Little did that innocent, smiling child know how life was about to change. Much to my grandmother's anguish, I was sent to boarding school at the age of six.

Attending boarding school meant that all my stuff now had to be clearly labelled, indicating ownership. Somehow, this applied another layer to my identity, yet simultaneously took away my freedom.

Further into boarding school attendance, I'm also seen on a rare weekend *exeat*, with Honey Bee in Nanny Win's garden, wearing my winter Sunday-best uniform. Other photographs show aspects of daily life – the gym, the library and the playing field – within the flint walls of Summerlea School.

At school there were few secrets. However, little did they know that in my young mind, the 'S' badge stitched onto my blazer pocket didn't represent Summerlea School, but Sarah. Me. My secret identity.

For a short while, the House Captain badge shone on my blazer, bright with optimism and responsibility, until the realisation dawned that with responsibility came a heaviness, an alienation. Resistance. I was only made House Captain the one time.

The Tufty Club started as a road-safety initiative for children in 1961, but went on to include home and water safety. In a place where I found it difficult to trust, Tufty and Willy Weasel were my special secret friends.

LOT **32**

## FIVE VINTAGE GLASS AND CERAMIC ORNAMENTS IN A GREY BOX

$0–$5

I can't say much about this motley crew, other than that they were my crew, who sat as neatly as they could on the dressing table, which neatly held all my neatly labelled uniforms in my neatly timetabled life at the neatly organised institution that was boarding school in the 1960s.

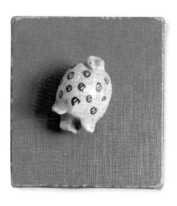
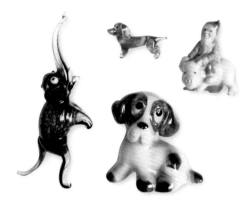

Battered, chipped and broken, they now squash together more comfortably and quietly in their grey home, the box that formerly contained the neatly on-time alarm clock that always started my neatly timetabled day.

LOT **33**

## VINTAGE MOROCCAN TOOLED-LEATHER MANICURE SET, INSCRIBED, MID-1960s, AND TIN OF FINGERNAIL CLIPPINGS

$5–$10

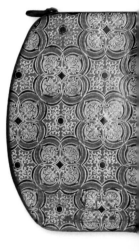

When I went to boarding school, my maternal grandmother presented me with this exotic red and golden leather-bound manicure set. It was such a treasure, such a thing of beauty and wonderment, and I had absolutely no idea what all the contents were to be used for. It intrigued me, terrified me, and made me feel special yet uncomfortable. It spoke of a world of which I had no knowledge, a world to which I somehow knew I would never comfortably belong – a grown-up woman's world.

At boarding school, we had to have clean hands and short, neat nails. To someone whose main pleasure was being in the open air, climbing trees and mucking around in the earth, this was a major challenge. In secondary school (still boarding), although we were allowed slightly longer nails, girls like me who took piano lessons were obliged to keep their nails short. So, when I left both boarding school and the dreaded piano lessons, I let those nails grow, grow, grow. I expressed my freedom by painting them all sorts of crazy colours and designs. They became an act of independence, of rebellion, of expression. So, I kept them. I keep these now, as they remind me of how, long ago, and in such a small way, my identity and my personality were being forged.

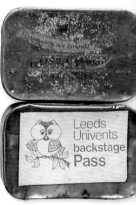

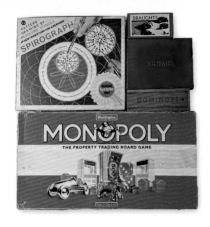

## LOT 34
## ASSORTED GAMES – DRAUGHTS, SOLITAIRE, DOMINOES, MONOPOLY AND SPIROGRAPH SET
$40–$60

The Spirograph set was my all-time favourite, a system that created all sorts of mandala-based patterns and designs. I was never much of a freehand sketcher, so I welcomed this 'toolkit'. It came with the traditional four coloured biro pens, all with especially long tips, designed to fit into the holes of the plastic circles and spheres – small components that I took great care not to lose. I searched and searched the stationery shops trying to find other long-tipped coloured pens. Alas, I was ahead of my time, as only red, blue, black and green were available.

It was hard to find people willing to sit down and play a long game of Monopoly with me. I loved Monopoly. The adrenaline would pump through my veins as I swiftly collected the brown rows of cheaper housing on the Old Kent Road and Whitechapel Road, which seemed more attainable than the exclusive royal blue Mayfair and Piccadilly. This was a time before gentrification, a phenomenon that, in my adult life, I have been a part of.

## LOT 35
## ASSORTED ITEMS INCLUDING A 'TOKEN' AND FOUR COINS, AND THREE PHOTOGRAPHS
$80–$100

In every aspect of my life I was a misfit. In 1962, when I was seven, my military parents chose not to live on an RAF camp, deciding instead to make the foray into the outside world of home-ownership by purchasing a newly built house at 10 Hawkes End in Brampton, Huntingdon in Cambridgeshire. Living off-camp meant that I had no opportunity to meet with similar kids – RAF kids who had also been sent away to boarding school, and with whom I might have forged friendships through that commonality during the school holidays. On this newly developing housing estate, the local kids had already made friends. I was an outsider, and having a private-school education did me no favours in their world.

My parents were both out at work all day, so during the school holidays, I was a 'latchkey kid'. Suffering from loneliness and boredom, I had to rely

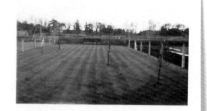

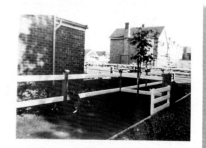

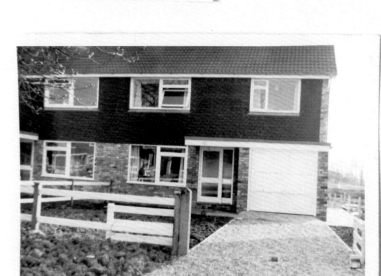

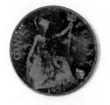

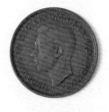

LOT **35**

on myself for entertainment. For quite some time after we had moved into our brand-new house, the back garden remained a huge muddy plot. My father had hired a rotovator, churning the heavy clay-based earth and uncovering fragments, which I eagerly gathered.

This became my private, personal playground, where another world slowly opened to me – a world of mystery, enquiry, fantasy and intrigue, as I uncovered relics from another time. The small cardboard box labelled 'Old Things' contains some of the treasures I found – a fragment of clay pipe, a miniature bottle stopper, a key, a squashed thimble. These objects fascinated me because of the stories I felt they could tell, and soon they became my very own talismans.

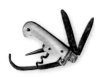

### LOT 36

### MINIATURE STEEL PENKNIFE WITH MOTHER-OF-PEARL CASING, c1900, BRITISH PASSPORT, DATE OF ISSUE 1996, PHOTOGRAPH, c1930, AND PUSH-OUT CARD OF A GIRL IN TROUSERS, WITH 'SARAH JANE' WRITTEN AT THE BASE
$40–$60

The photograph shows my grandmother, Nanny Win, in a tree. During the school holidays, I spent much of my time alone. Away from the constrictions of an all-girl boarding school, I revelled in the freedom of activities that included climbing trees, exploring the building site of the new housing estate where we lived and digging in the soil looking for stuff. People said I took after my grandmother, who grew up riding and tending horses, and doing a lot of physical labour. I had a short haircut, found boy's clothes much more comfortable and identified as neither a girl nor a boy. I was, simply, me. That is, until one day I was alone, hanging upside-down on the parallel bars in the local playing fields, when a group of older boys approached me, asking, "Are you a boy or a girl?"

As I looked down, I saw this miniature penknife glinting in the grass beneath my head. I dropped off the bars, hastily picked up and pocketed the knife, and answered, "A girl, why?"

"Prove it," the biggest boy smirked. I ran – so fast. I scarpered, didn't look back, not really understanding why or how, but I knew that this was not a good situation to be in, and in that moment a new-found awareness was thrust upon me.

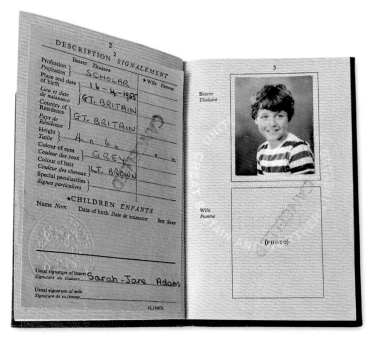

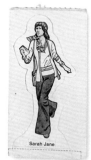

Sarah Jane

The newly acquired lucky penknife tucked in my pocket immediately became a symbol of protection, an emblem of courage, and a question and confirmation of identity to me.

## LOT 37

## COLLECTION OF FOUNTAIN PENS, INCLUDING A PARKER AND SHEAFFER, AND INK BOTTLES, c1960

$50–$80

In the 1960s, when children had learnt to write with a pencil, their progression was not to the biro, but to the fountain pen. Owning a fountain pen was a rite of passage, signalling a move towards adulthood. It was impossible to erase something written with a fountain pen, so thoughts had to be clearly defined prior to committing them to paper.

I wasn't sure I liked this idea and, although I loved my pen, even the exotic bright-turquoise ink I was allowed to use didn't lessen the trepidation I felt when putting pen to paper. Decades later, at primary school in Australia, my children seemed to share the same feelings on receiving their 'pen licence'.

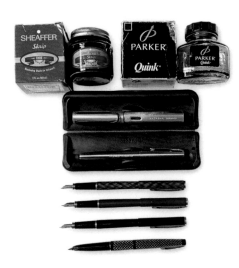

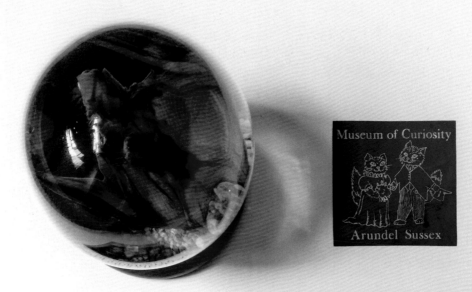

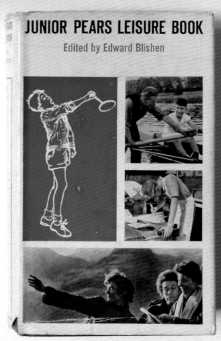

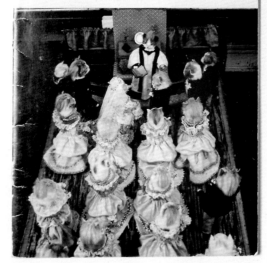

POTTER'S MUSEUM
OF CURIOSITY

6 HIGH STREET, ARUNDEL, SUSSEX

Museum of Curiosity

Arundel  Sussex

JUNIOR PEARS LEISURE BOOK

Edited by Edward Blishen

LOT **38**

## *JUNIOR PEARS LEISURE BOOK*, 1965, BROCHURE
## FROM POTTER'S MUSEUM OF CURIOSITY, PERSPEX BAT
## DOORSTOP, c1980, AND STICKER

$20–$30

These two publications represent the stark contrast between the life it was hoped and encouraged that I would lead and an alternative world of weird curiosities that totally mesmerised and fascinated me. The dichotomy did not go unnoticed, even when I was little.

The former, which I was given when I was 10, is a neatly turned-out book full of images of well-scrubbed, rosy-cheeked people happily playing outdoor games, sports and other group activities. It remains unopened and unread on my bookshelf.

The latter describes an incredible collection of taxidermy in Arundel, which, as a youngster, I visited numerous times. Undoubtedly this museum, a veritable 'Cabinet of Curiosities', was a massive enlightenment – a light-bulb moment and inspiration for a young girl who had never had an affinity with the world around her. Alongside Potter's 'fantastic' dioramas, the museum held a number of other curiosities – deformed animals, such as a two-headed kitten and a chicken with four legs, and relics from other cultures and times.

Walter Potter was an Englishman who lived from the 1800s until the early 1900s in Bramber in rural Sussex. He was a self-taught taxidermist, who for some 60 years, stuffed, dressed, bejewelled and presented small animals in a series of scenes and pastiches, including 'Who Killed Cock Robin?', 'The Kittens' Tea & Croquet Party', 'The Kittens' Wedding', 'The Upper Ten' and 'The Lower Five', which formed the core of the museum exhibit. When the museum was forced to close, visionary artist Damien Hirst tried to purchase the entire collection for one million pounds. Sadly, however, the collection was broken up and sold off in lots at an auction by Bonhams in 2003.

The doorstop, which I acquired in a market much later in life, is a real bat preserved in a perspex sphere.

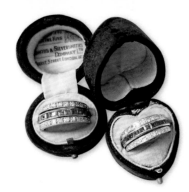

## LOT 39

## TWO 18CT WHITE-GOLD TRIPLE ETERNITY RINGS COMPRISING A CENTRAL BAND OF DIAMONDS WITH HALF HOOP OF SAPPHIRE AND RUBY HINGED ON EITHER SIDE, BOXED, c1920

$3000–$3500

When I was about 10 years old, my mother and her sister's families spent time together. One day, my younger cousin was admiring my mother's engagement ring and playing with her accompanying swivel eternity ring. That fascinating ring, made in the 1920s, had a central full-circle of diamonds on which either side were set, in two hinged half hoops, a row of sapphires and a row of rubies. The ring could be worn in three different combinations and we girls were delighted by its ingenuity.

My cousin expressed her love of my mother's two most precious pieces, whereby my mother promised them to her. I remember feeling sick to the stomach. Although I had no understanding of the items' monetary value, their preciousness represented something else, in which, it seemed, I was not included.

As an adult working in the antique jewellery trade, I rarely came across such pieces. So, when two rings turned up at different times and locations, I couldn't part with them and still today, have two triple eternity rings. One for me and one for my twin sister.

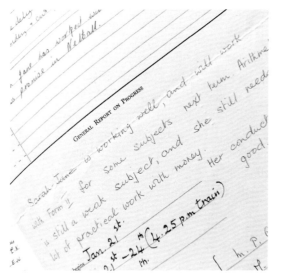

## LOT 40

## SCHOOL REPORTS FROM SUMMERLEA SCHOOL, 1963

NCV

Maths: "Arithmetic is still a weak subject and she still needs a lot of practical work with money."

Art: "Sarah Jane works with enthusiasm and has a nice sense of colour."

Music: "Sarah Jane is able to do the work but does not always contribute helpfully in class."

| | | | |
|---|---|---|---|
| B | sometimes lack ... | | |
| ...ICS } | C | Fairly good. Sarah-Jane works with interest and enthusiasm. | JC. |
| ...RY | C | Quite good. Sarah-Jane has worked with interest ... | |
| | | Sarah-Jane works with enthusiasm and has a nice sense of colour | JC. |
| | | Sarah-Jane is able to do the work but does not always contribute helpfully in class. | J.O.Y. |

| | | | |
|---|---|---|---|
| | | ...ome is lively and interested in class and has produced some good work. I had hoped for a better examination result. | 42 |
| | | | JS. |
| | B | Sarah Jane's work has been excellent. | AM. | 74 |
| | | Good. Sarah-Jane has continued to work well both in class and preparation; she has some original ideas. J.O.Y | 73 |

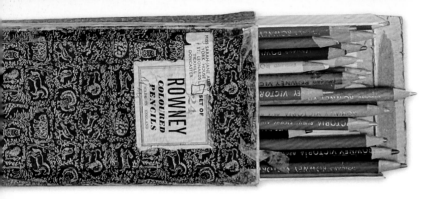

## LOT 41
### BOX OF ROWNEY COLOURING PENCILS, IN ORIGINAL BOX, c1970
$5–$10

The box of Rowney coloured pencils was my first serious box of crayons. Although I could copy a map from the blackboard faster than anyone else, and could trace, colour in and copy neatly and efficiently, I was totally useless at imaginative drawing. Therefore, these beauties, my pride and joy, got very little use. However, I adored the colours and spent plenty of time 'sorting them out' – lining up colours from light to dark, grading their hues, experimenting with ways they could be blended together, shading colours together and separately, and playing with saturation. I was happiest when they were neatly lined up in their box, all sharpened, with perfect colour grading. I can't begin to tell you how irritated I became when, due to the leads breaking and their consequent sharpening, the crayons' lengths didn't correlate with the grading of the colours.

## LOT 42
### BOX OF CHARCOALS AND LINO-CUTTING TOOL SET, c1970
$5–$10

The best part of lino-cutting was the smell of the linseed oil, which was a component of the lino squares we were given to work with. I found it nigh impossible to work in reverse – imagining a negative-positive of an image just didn't resonate in my brain. I generally ended up frustrated and with injuries to my hands as a result of not being interested, hence the completeness and great condition of this set of tools.

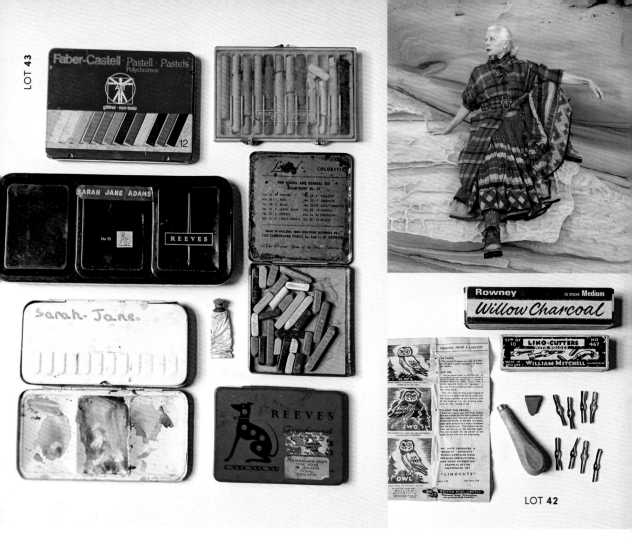

LOT **42**

## LOT **43**
## **MIXED LOT OF WATERCOLOUR PAINTS AND COLOURED PASTELS, c1970**
$30–$40

Despite my love of colour and the encouragement of the gorgeously shaped blue paint tins, which cleverly opened out to provide a triptych palette for mixing, I never progressed as an imaginative creative painter. I preferred collage, using pre-existing materials to create textural, layered work. I was developing a feel for medium- and pattern-mixing, working with scraps I'd gathered rather than starting from scratch – definitely a recycler rather than a new designer.

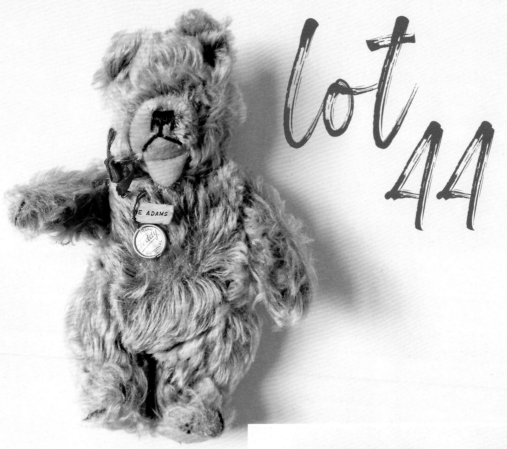

lot
44

The overwhelming sense
of abandonment.
trepidation and
disappointment I felt
meant that even now
I am notoriously early
when checking in
for flights.

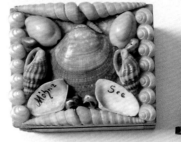

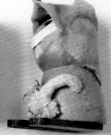

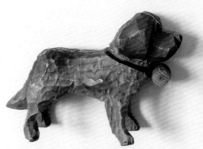

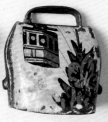

LOT 45

## LOT 44

## 'TEDDY-HERMANN' TEDDY BEAR WITH
## ORIGINAL LABEL, c1967

$80–$100

My father was posted to Germany, the birthplace of Teddy-Hermann, and he gave me this deluxe teddy bear when I started at my secondary boarding school, aged 12. I'm sad to confess that I never felt the same love for Hermann as I did for my little Tessie (Lot 21). There are no signs of a life lived on his cheerful tight face – no eyes missing, all fur intact. Poor Hermann, he remains in perfect condition to this day – untouched, unsullied, unloved.

## LOT 45

## FOUR SOUVENIRS FROM GERMANY
## AND SWITZERLAND, 1966–1969

$10–$20

In 1967, I changed boarding schools, moving from Sussex to Hertfordshire for my secondary education. During the school holidays, I was to fly from England to Germany, where my father was based on an RAF station near München Gladbach (now Mönchengladbach). For my first ever flight, at 12 years of age, my aunt and uncle were asked to collect me from boarding school and drop me at Gatwick airport, where I was to fly unaccompanied on a charter flight to Germany. At the end of term, I was the last child to be collected. The traffic to the airport was bad and consequently I missed the flight. I don't know how it happened, but I ended up making the journey in an RAF military aircraft, sitting in a row along the side of an aeroplane full of men dressed in full military fatigues. The overwhelming sense of abandonment, trepidation and disappointment I felt meant that even now I am notoriously early when checking in for flights.

During those summer holidays, my parents and I went on a three-week camping trip from Germany through Switzerland and down to Italy. This, and many other trips, is recorded in my 'Exploring' journal (Lot 46). These souvenirs are one from each trip made.

The carved wooden St Bernard dog was purchased in 1967 from a souvenir shop at the top of the Great St Bernard Pass. The handpainted cow bell is a souvenir from the summer of 1968, where, "smashing south", as my father described it, we stopped in Salzburg to explore the salt mines and cable cars, before heading through the Dolomites, a picture-perfect area where the hills were truly alive with the sound of music; that is, the 'tong-tong-tong' of the cow bells (DH Lawrence, *The Captain's Doll*, 1923).

## LOT 46
### CHILD'S TRAVEL JOURNAL TITLED, 'EXPLORING', 1966–1969
$80–$100

This journal consists of 160 pages of handwritten tales, with more than 100 postcards and other mementos from travels that I was taken on between the age of 11 and 15. Being based in Germany meant ready access to the rest of Europe and, as my father was a lover of driving, school holidays were spent touring through Germany, Holland, Austria, Italy and Switzerland. I would collect postcards and paraphernalia along the way

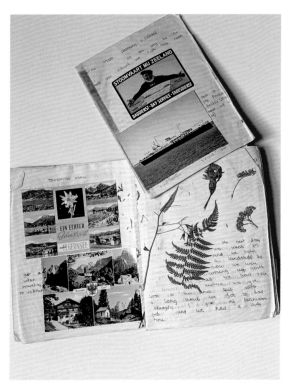

– entry tickets, sweet packets, menus and brochures. Every evening, rather than going to play with the other kids in the campsite, I had to sit in our tent and write about the day's events in this journal. It offers glimpses of our family-holiday life, which seemed to revolve mainly around visiting as many ancient sites, wartime memorials and museums as possible.

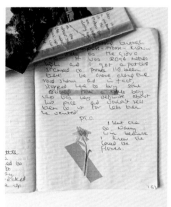

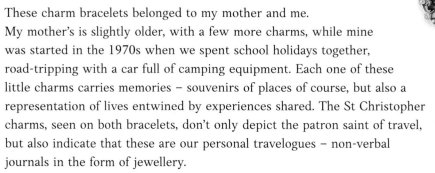

## LOT **47**
## **TWO SILVER CHARM BRACELETS, c1965–1970**

$200–$300

These charm bracelets belonged to my mother and me.
My mother's is slightly older, with a few more charms, while mine
was started in the 1970s when we spent school holidays together,
road-tripping with a car full of camping equipment. Each one of these
little charms carries memories – souvenirs of places of course, but also a
representation of lives entwined by experiences shared. The St Christopher
charms, seen on both bracelets, don't only depict the patron saint of travel,
but also indicate that these are our personal travelogues – non-verbal
journals in the form of jewellery.

During the months before our trips, my father would pore over maps
planning the route. It became something akin to a military exercise – a
'recce' – as places of interest were added, prioritised or removed from
the plan. My mother was in charge of the camp kitchen, stocking up on
non-perishables for easy-to-cook, two-pan meals, along with a medicine kit.
These trips were a major operation.

I would sit in the back of the car, squashed in amongst the pillows,
blankets and all the paraphernalia that family life on the road in the 1960s
required. They were happy days. For our arrival at the designated camping
site, we had quickly streamlined the set-up for efficiency. The giant frame
of the tent would be constructed, with the props set at half height. My role
was to stand, doubled over, in the middle of the frame, with the heavy
canvas tent on my back. My parents would then systematically unfold
the tent, tie the corners and raise the roof, and our home would take shape.

Incredible really, to think that so many personal memories are
encapsulated in these two versions of the gazillions of charm bracelets
that were collected during these times.

*non-verbal journals in the form of jewellery*

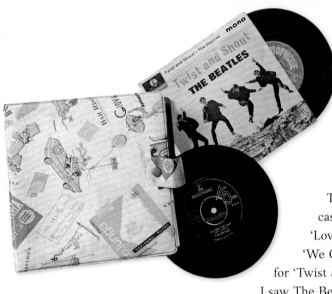

## LOT 48
### VINYL RECORD CASE, c1960, WITH 20 ASSORTED 45RPM RECORDS
$200–$300

This touring-holiday-inspired record case includes The Beatles' recordings of 'Love me Do', 'Can't Buy Me Love' and 'We Can Work It Out', and an empty sleeve for 'Twist and Shout'.

I saw The Beatles for the first time in 1964, on the black-and-white television that took pride of place in my uncle's recently modernised home. They were performing 'Twist and Shout', and it was a life-changing moment. I remember the (male) grown-ups in the household shouting to the women in the kitchen, "Come and look at this lot! Look at their hair!"

As far as I was allowed, I grew a Beatles mop whilst saving my pocket money to buy my first single, 'Twist and Shout'. When I had saved enough, my parents suggested that I spend the money "wisely" on a long-playing record album recorded by some random cover group. I was mortified at the thought, and rejected it immediately, as I knew I wanted the original. Not much has changed. Authenticity all the way, baby.

## LOT 49
### THREE AUTOGRAPH BOOKS, 1967–1969
$500–$600

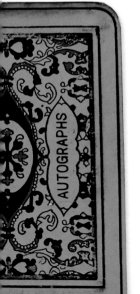

One of these autograph books includes signatures of many Formula One motor racing drivers, including those shown here: Jim Clark and Jack Brabham. Other signatures include Graham Hill, Jackie Oliver, Jackie Stewart, Jochen Rindt, Alan Rees and Jacky Ickx.

During our European road trips, we visited numerous ancient monuments and old buildings, as well as attending motor-racing events. In my 'Exploring' journal of 1967 (Lot 46), I cover a three-week camping holiday, when we drove as far south as Pompeii in Italy. Our first stop was Nürburgring to attend the German Grand Prix. We pitched our tent at the Jakobs-Muhle

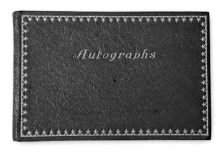

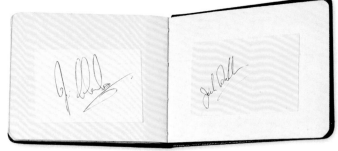

campsite, near the race track. There, I met a lady named Ann, who was working with the David Hobbs crew. She very kindly took my bright, shiny new autograph book and my collection of famous autographs began.

Over the course of that time I was questioning whether I should have been born a boy. I frequently felt a sense of disassociation and found a way to entertain myself by following motorsport, my favourite driver being the Belgian, Jacky Ickx.

## LOT 50

### RAF OFFICER'S CAP AND UNUSED RAF FLYING OVERALLS, PRIVATE PILOT'S LICENCE AND MEDICAL RECORDS, VARIOUS DATES

$30–$50

At work, my father was either dressed in flying overalls, or in formal RAF uniform (mess kit). I sensed his pride and excitement when dressed in the overalls, yet when he was in his mess kit, he seemed uncomfortably restricted, despite the respect the uniform commanded. I felt that underneath he yearned to be free, to be himself.

In his spare time, mainly spent alone in his garage restoring old motorbikes and cars, my father's 'uniform' was very old, tattered, comfortable clothes, generally stained, worn and faded.

My choice of dress, like my father's, is a rebellion against the rules imposed by the formality of a uniform that also contained me for so much of my childhood.

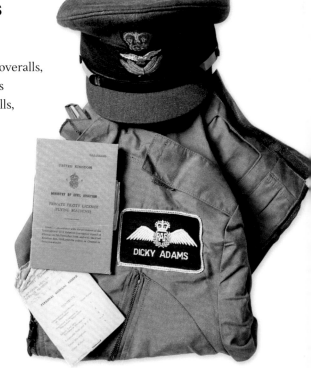

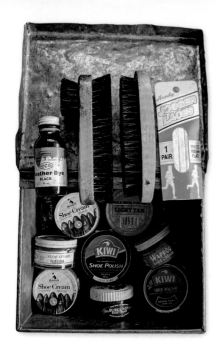

## LOT 51
### TIN BOX WITH SHOE-SHINING IMPLEMENTS
$5–$10

I remember my grandfather sitting on an old stool out the back in a singlet and working trousers, vigorously polishing his heavy black leather boots. The rhythmical movement of the brush, the wonderful smell of the polish and the reflective black shine that was revealed in the process were all so satisfying to watch. He had an added technique, 'spit and polish', which he told me he had learnt during wartime when he was in the army.

At boarding school, Saturday morning was timetabled for shoe-polishing duty, and I would think of Grandpa whilst performing this task, which somehow had become a drudge. The dark tan polish got stuck in the punched-out design holes and buckles of my brown leather sandals. It would get everywhere – on my school dress, around my fingernails and too much on the cloth. How easily had one man's pride become a young girl's frustration.

Despite my youthful failings, I always maintained my shoes and, later, my battered and worn black leather jacket. The supple, wrinkled and creased leather jacket – the first 'luxury' I purchased for myself as a young punk – represented strength, toughness, fearlessness and revolution. I knew I could depend on it to keep me covered and protected.

## LOT 52
### HANDPAINTED ENAMEL ON SILVER BROOCH, c1900, *THE REAL ISADORA*, BY VICTOR SEROFF (HUTCHINSON), 1972, AND ASSORTED PHOTOGRAPHS, c1969
$600–$800

My mother decided to have some professional photographs taken and she brought me along. I found it exceedingly uncomfortable that the photographer seemed extremely interested in taking these shots of me in ridiculously staged dress-ups.

Later, one of my teenage role models was American-born dancer and choreographer Isadora Duncan (1877–1927), who sadly lost her life when

# lot 52

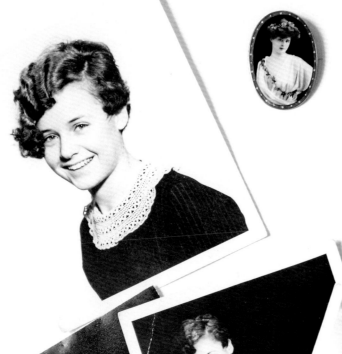

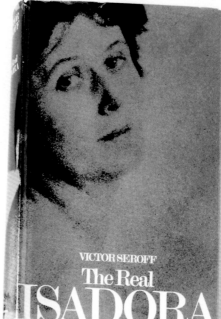

VICTOR SEROFF
The Real
ISADORA

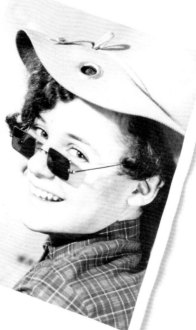

the long, flowing silk scarf she was wearing became entangled in the spoked wheel of an open-topped sports car. I devoured every book written about this fascinating woman. Isadora was a free-spirited bohemian, an atheist, a communist, an artist. She had two illegitimate children, never wore jewellery and became a total inspiration as to how I intended to live my life as a free spirit.

The brooch has been in my collection for decades, and this Edwardian beauty, an Isadora look-alike, is also an inspiration to me (see Lot 76).

## LOT 53
## PIECE OF ENGRAVED WHITE STONE, AND COLOUR PHOTOGRAPH, c1969
NCV (WITHDRAWN)

I picked up this stone on a beach in Gaeta, Italy. I have no idea what it was used for, although the scored circumference makes me wonder if it was a bottle stopper or possibly used in some way with fishing nets. Any information would be gratefully received. It will stay with me until the riddle is solved. This is also pretty much the first and last time I wore a bikini. I was uncomfortable with my sexuality and the lack of freedom that wearing this ridiculous garment afforded me.

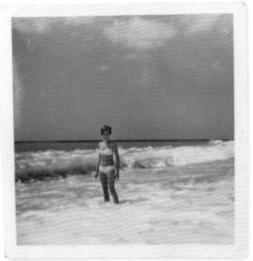

*This is the first and last time I wore a bikini.*

## LOT **54**

## **FIVE COPIES OF** *OZ***, 1972, NINE COPIES OF** *i-D***, 1985, AND ASSORTED PUNK MAGAZINES**

$100–$130

At boarding school breakfast time, after we had recited grace, the BBC News would be played over the loudspeaker. No conversation was allowed until both these rituals had been completed. News of obscenity trials against the editors of the underground magazine *OZ* quietly motivated the 16-year-old me to obtain copies of the magazine. When I did, they felt like an entry ticket into a grown-up and subversive world that I was secretly and tentatively trying to explore.

At around this time, I had also written letters (sent from school) to the Young Communist League (YCL). We were not allowed to receive phone calls at school, so I was in shock when I was pulled from class one morning to take a telephone call in the principal's office. I assumed I was about to receive some dreadful news. This feeling was compounded when I discovered who was at the other end of the line – a representative of YCL. The principal listened to the entire call and somehow I survived the fall-out. That was the beginning – and swift end – of my overtly political career. I decided there and then that quiet subversion, questionable disruption and counter-revolution by more subtle and ambiguous ways would be my method. I continue to use this method of communicating my beliefs and opinions to this day. Underground and coded.

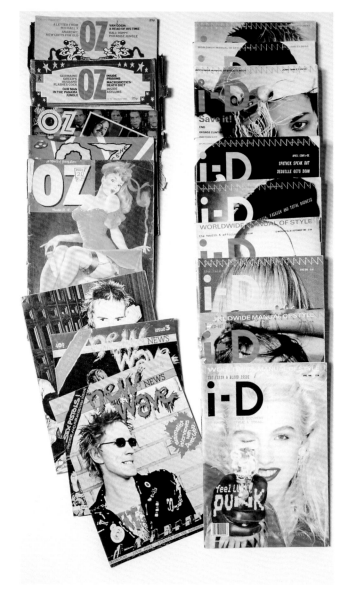

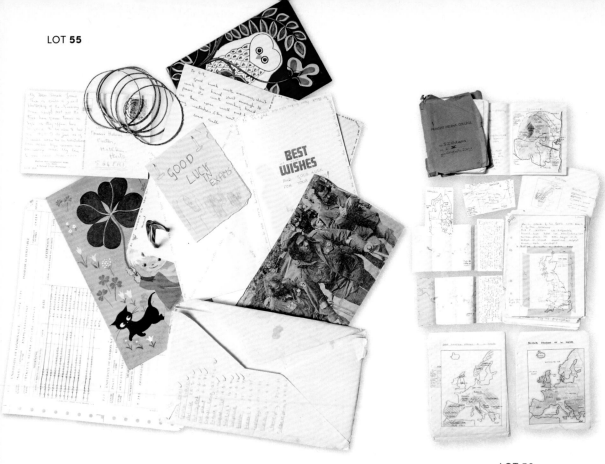

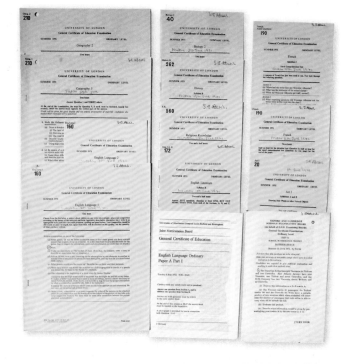

Geography, English
Language, Biology,
History, Religious
Knowledge, English
Literature, French, Art,
Mathematics.

## LOT 55

## COLLECTION OF SILVER BANGLES, TRADITIONAL AFRICAN SILVER V RING, AND ASSORTED CARDS AND PAPERS, 1971

$70–$100

At 16, I was stuck in an all-girls boarding school. Surrounded by, yet terribly isolated from, the other girls – although all of us were to a greater or lesser degree in the same situation. We were about to take our 'O' (ordinary) level exams and I was signed up to sit nine subjects. The sense of despair, panic, stress and loneliness was making me physically ill. Unlike many of the girls whose 'privileged' futures were already determined – futures that included finishing school, debutante balls and entry into high society – yours truly needed to do well academically.

Clearly, on a 'good luck in your exams' card, one school friend shared my thoughts, writing: "Don't get too depressed and think how lucky you are getting out of this dump."

The set of silver bangles was my first-ever jewellery trade. I had swapped them a few years earlier with a fellow student at the boarding school.

The silver V ring is one of my most treasured pieces. A traditional African wedding ring, it was brought from Nigeria especially for me by a fellow student and friend, Chinwe Dike. Chinwe, the daughter of the ambassador to the short-lived Republic of Biafra, was the only girl of colour at our boarding school. On the day the BBC morning news announced the tragic and sudden death of Jimi Hendrix, Chinwe left the table and ran sobbing from the refectory. I so respected her for courageously displaying her overwhelming grief and envied the freedom she showed by this passionate outburst of emotion.

## LOT 56

## COLLECTION OF CUE CARDS AND NINE 'O' LEVEL EXAM PAPERS, JOINT MATRICULATION BOARD (JMB) CENTRAL CERTIFICATE OF EDUCATION, 1971

$5–$10

Geography, English Language, Biology, History, Religious Knowledge, English Literature, French, Art, Mathematics.

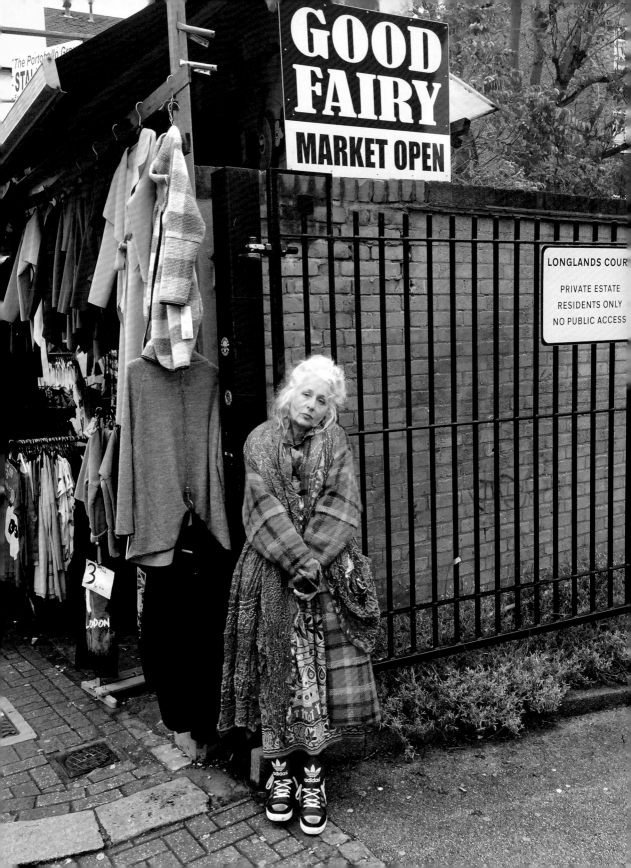

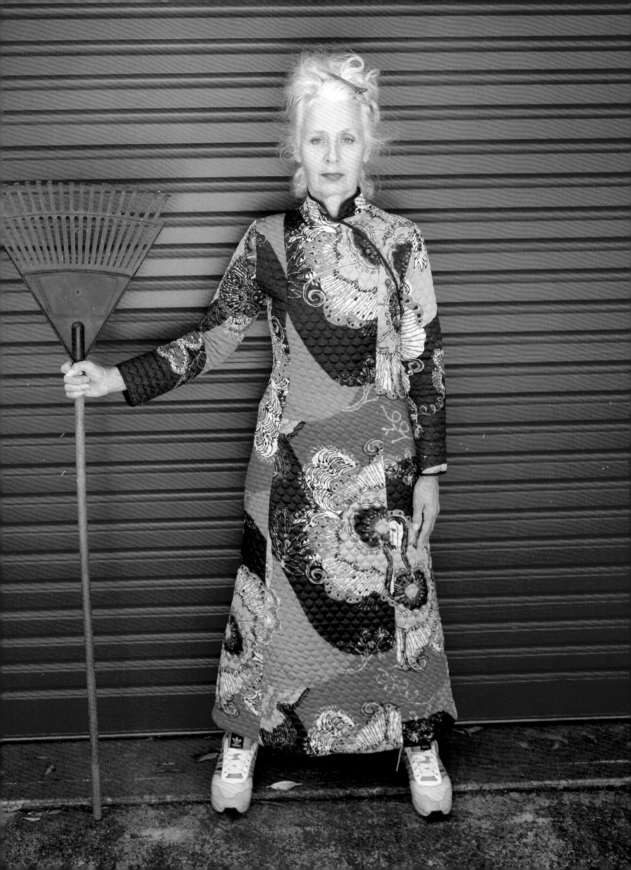

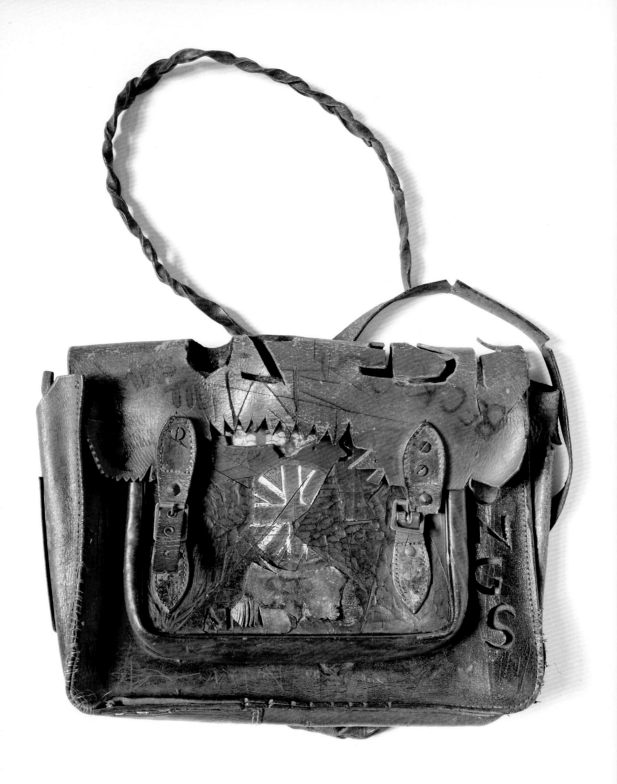

LOT **59**

# my ride to independence

## LOT 57

## GLASS 'MOTORCYCLE' SCENT BOTTLE, c1930, AND SCHOOL REPORTS, 1973

$80–$120

My parents had left Germany and bought a newly built house on a small housing estate in Tickhill, a quaint village in Yorkshire. My mother rather grandly named it York House, supposedly because there were some lumps of locally quarried sandstone in the back garden. As southerners, this was something of a novelty. I always found the name pretentious and embarrassing, and the locals must have thought we were a right bunch of wankers.

I had indicated to my parents that if they wanted me to complete 'A' level studies, I wanted to leave private school. I think they were surprised when their threat of my attendance at the local comprehensive school was gleefully received.

My father was stationed at RAF Bawtry, and my mother was working in Doncaster as a PA at the National Coal Board. My interview with the principal at Maltby Comprehensive School was scheduled on a day they were both working, and public transport was intermittent at best.

I had never driven a motorbike or car, but my father (an RAF flying instructor) gave me a crash course in motorbike riding. My first solo ride was along the winding country roads between Tickhill and Maltby – to my school interview.

The principal, knowing I was fresh out of a Home Counties boarding school, was taken aback when I turned up dressed in full leathers, with a motorcycle helmet under my arm. The interview went well and I was offered a place at the school.

My excitement quickly abated, though, when I returned to the car park to find the bike on its side. I must not have secured the stand correctly. The thing was so heavy that I couldn't raise it. I had to wait hours for someone to help, during which time I was worried sick that the bike had suffered damage on its underside. Fortunately, it was unscathed and my late return home went unnoticed.

So began my new life, and this scent bottle reminds me of the day I started my long ride to independence.

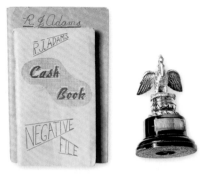

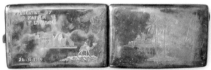

## LOT **58**
### PAPERWEIGHT, 1959, AND SILVER CIGARETTE CASE DATED 26 NOVEMBER 1960
$80–$150

After so long away, I was finally living full-time with my parents. I felt like an invader in their life, a stranger in their home. The paperweight sat in pride of place on their sideboard. The silver cigarette case was found in my father's 'Life in a Box'. It depicts the Taq Kasra, an ancient brickwork arch, which is the only monument remaining from the 2nd- to 7th-century city of Ctesiphon, Persia. I understand this cigarette case was a special gift presented to him by an Iraqi student on the event of his 'passing out' (graduation) in 1960.

## LOT **59**
### LEATHER SCHOOL SATCHEL, 1972
$10–$20 (WITHDRAWN)

This was the year I first fell in love – not only with life, but also with a boy. He was a local in the year above me at Maltby Comprehensive School. Not too long after I'd started there, he stopped me in the corridor, blurting out that he thought he was in love with me. Michael was intense and passionate, and we quickly became obsessed with one another. A small but gangly lad with long straight hair and freckles, he was also an incredibly talented artist and photographer, with a way of looking at the world that was different, which somehow I understood. I would visit him at his home, a tiny back-to-back worker's cottage on the top of the ridge in Maltby – a far cry from York House in Tickhill. Here, under the strange darkroom lights in his tiny bedroom, we lost both ourselves and our virginity.

He gave me his school satchel, already heavily customised – 'distressed' with carvings, graffiti and plaited leather straps. This gift, from my first love, is one of my most treasured possessions. The guitar strings were used later to repair where the stitching is missing.

## EDWARDIAN 9CT GOLD AND AMETHYST RING IN BOX, AND SELECTED FOSSILS AND EPHEMERA INCLUDING 'A' LEVEL GEOLOGY NOTES

$120–$150

My 'A' level subjects were Geology, Geography, English and General Studies. One of the marvellous things about studying geology and geography was going on field trips. We were herded onto buses that transported us to spectacular locations throughout Yorkshire. For the first time in my life, I was hanging out with boys and, oh my, it was fun. They seemed so much more straightforward than the girls I'd been at school with. Housed in basic accommodation for two or three nights, we larked about, pulling and pushing one another in all weathers, whilst trudging up and down muddy hillsides, digging for fossils, collecting specimens and drawing examples of rock formations.

The field trips combined both years of 'A' level students, so my artist boyfriend, who was also studying geography, came along on the trip to Malham Cove in the Yorkshire Dales National Park. The notes and sketches of limestone shown here are his work. The doodles are mine; the words, ours.

Back in the classroom, the study of rocks and minerals, crystallography, was logical, practical, clear, enduring and beautiful. I experienced a deep sense of contentment; I was exhilarated and fulfilled.

The amethyst ring was the first gift a boy had ever bought for me. When she saw it, my mother was horrified, asking me, "Have you got engaged?"

I guess we sort of had.

*The amethyst ring was the first gift a boy had ever bought for me.*

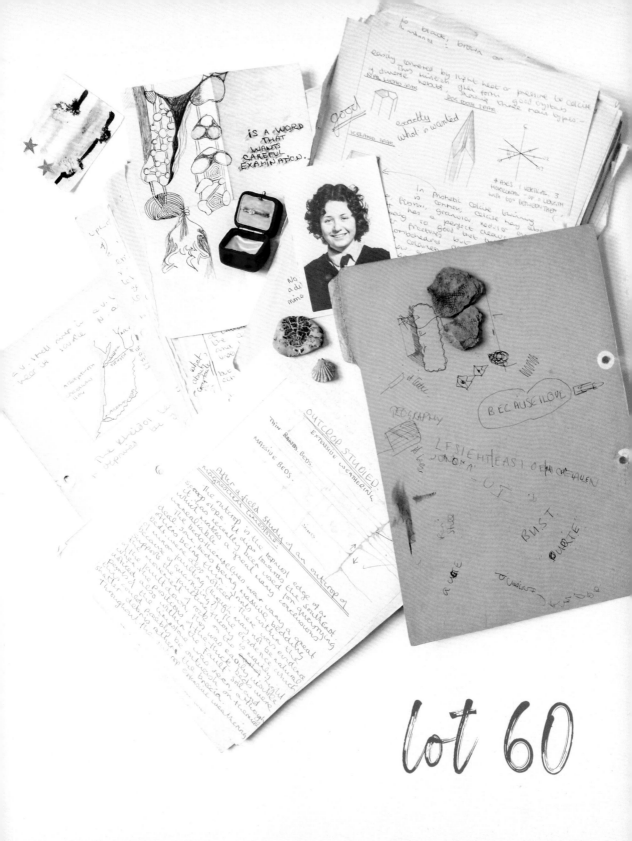

lot 60

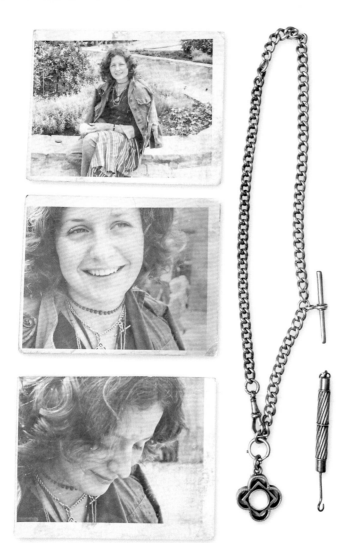

## LOT 61
### SILVER ALBERT CHAIN WITH COMPASS FOB AND PROPELLING GLOVE HOOK, EARLY 1900s, AND THREE PHOTOGRAPHS, 1973
$250–$280

On weekends, my boyfriend and I would visit different cities throughout Yorkshire to go to galleries where he'd be exhibiting. We'd travel miles on the bus, often with oil paintings on huge canvases. We would then explore, seeking out the second-hand stores and flea markets.

He had an amazing way of dressing, frequently going out in paint-splattered overalls or bright-yellow flared 'loon' pants teamed with painted red boots. In the photographs, his army jacket is draped around my shoulders and my candy-striped blazer (a nod to Rod Stewart) is over my leg. Together, we were an eyeful.

I was becoming more and more interested in antique jewellery, buying little pieces here and there. This Victorian Albert chain, compass fob and silver propelling glove hook had belonged to Nanny Win's mother.

The brass 'three wise monkeys' I'm wearing in the photos were hung on a length of leather and, along with the African coloured glass beads, are long gone.

This was one of the happiest times of my life. I was free to express myself and dress as I pleased, and I made the most of that freedom.

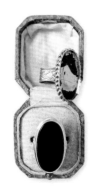

## LOT **62**

### ONYX RING SET IN 18CT GOLD, IN BOX, c1970, AND BASE METAL RING (STONE MISSING), c1960

$150–$180

I am fond of an oval-shaped ring. I bought this flat, low-set onyx ring, for £14 on one of our weekend sorties in Yorkshire. I wore it constantly – the smooth reflective black surface of the onyx was satisfying to me.

The oval metal ring had been given to me by my mother some time earlier. It had held a cabochon pink glass 'stone', which at the time seemed magical. Unfortunately, it was only glued into the cheap setting and one day it fell out and was lost. I got into so much trouble – and I never wore mass-produced jewellery again.

## LOT **63**

### LEATHER WRISTBAND, COPY OF WILLIAM SHAKESPEARE'S *MEASURE FOR MEASURE*, AND OTHER EPHEMERA

NCV (WITHDRAWN)

My second year at Maltby Comprehensive brought heartbreak and joy. My boyfriend had left school and was now attending art college. This separation meant that our love affair was unsustainable and we parted ways.

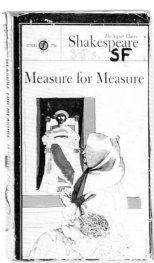

My second love, equally as strong, was a lad in the same year as me. He'd caught my attention because he had the longest hair in the school. Stephen Fellows was a musician – quiet, moody, intense, fragile and passionate. We shared a love of underground music, progressive (prog) rock, Marc Bolan and guitar solos. Yet again, my parents were horrified.

On weekends, I would catch the bus to go and watch him rehearsing with his band, Mrs Tibbitts. I'd perch on giant bags of potatoes in the storage space of the supermarket owned by the drummer's dad.

My boyfriend, together with the drummer, went on to have some success in the post-punk era in another band, The Comsat Angels. Many years later, when a band he was managing, the Little Glitches, played at the Enmore Theatre in Sydney,

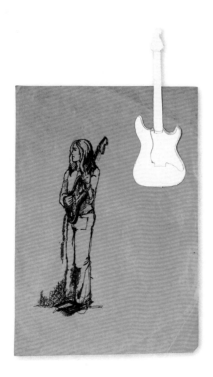
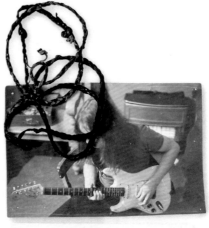
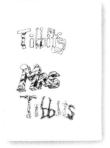
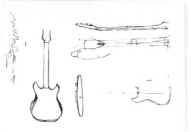
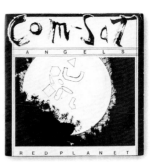

I delivered some of the trinkets he had given to me to a roadie, with a request that he return them to my former love. I felt perhaps he would appreciate having some of those tangibles back in his life, knowing that for me also, the past never changes. Those items included pins made for Mrs Tibbitts, along with some more leather bracelets. I hope he reads this and discovers that I am still 'Forever Young'.

The ink drawing of a boy playing a Stratocaster, together with the leather wristband (which you can see in the 2005 photograph of me in Lot 202), were gifts from him that I retained. The song is forever in my heart.

## LOT **64**

## FOUR 'A' LEVEL PAPERS, JMB CENTRAL CERTIFICATE OF EDUCATION, 1973

$5–$10

I took to geology and geography like a duck to water. I adored the study of rocks, fossils, people and places. Our 'A' level teachers were phenomenal – true mentors, with a knowledge and a passion for their subjects, the like of which I had never experienced before. I began to feel a sense of direction, an engagement, both with the people and topics, and the methods of study.

I won the Geography prize in my final year of school, but rather than attending the ceremony, where presentations were to be made by World War II flying hero Sir Douglas Bader, I opted to spend the week with my musician boyfriend and his family in a caravan in Bridlington, a coastal holiday town in Yorkshire. My parents missed their one and only motivation for visiting the school and I was never forgiven.

Whilst I achieved good results in my 'A' levels, because my musician boyfriend would be attending Sheffield College of Art, I disappointed my parents again by accepting a place at Sheffield University, rather than going to Oxford or Cambridge. My first-year subjects were Psychology, Sociology and Philosophy.

## LOT **65**

## **COLLECTION OF STATIONERY, c1973**

$1–$5

For my time between leaving school and starting university, rather than having a gap year, my mother organised a 10-week job for me, working as a casual in the National Coal Board.

This was wonderful, as I learnt so much. I learnt how to waste time. I learnt that I would never, ever again work in an office environment. I learnt to get over my addiction to stationery. I learnt of the brain-numbing effect of sniffing Snopake thinners, an addiction that stayed with me for some years.

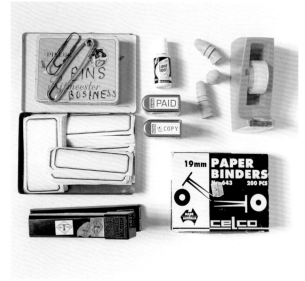

I learnt how to pretend to look busy. I learnt, with horror, the salacious ways that adults flirt. I learnt how to play the game. I learnt first-hand in the real world about social climbing.

I learnt that I wanted out of here – and fast.

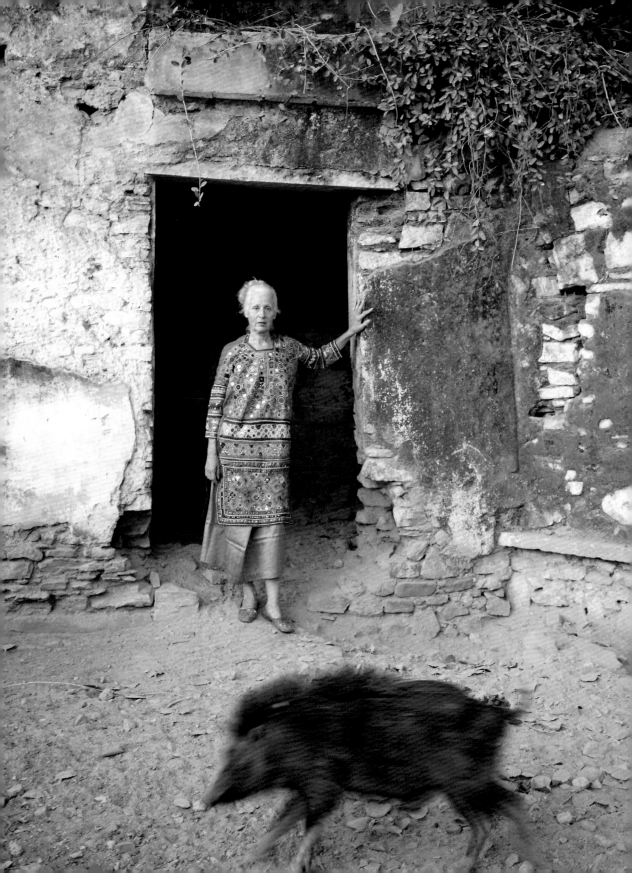

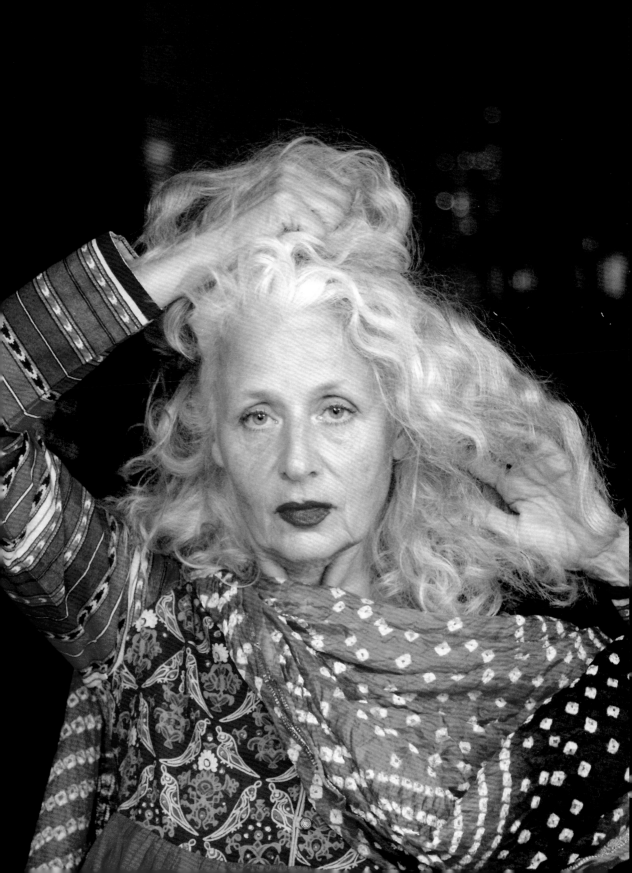

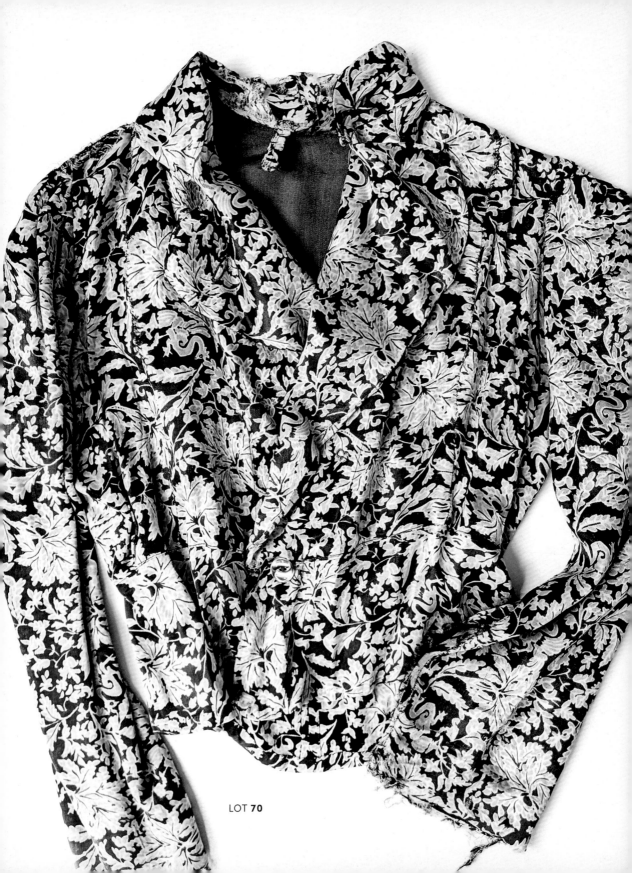

LOT **70**

# link to another life

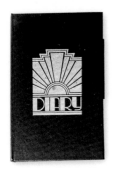

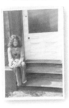

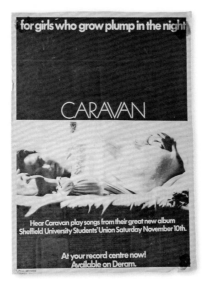

for girls who grow plump in the night

CARAVAN

Hear Caravan play songs from their great new album
Sheffield University Students' Union Saturday November 10th.

At your record centre now!
Available on Deram.

LOT **66**

## BIBA DIARY (PARTIALLY WRITTEN), 1974, AND GREEN CERAMIC MUG, c1970, AND CARAVAN ALBUM POSTER

$10–$30

Finally, I was free! A small load of belongings was delivered to Sheffield, where I had found my very own room in a large, once grand, now welcomingly dilapidated Victorian house. The room was already painted a dusky dark pink and was sparsely furnished with a bed, a table and a chair. I decorated it with posters, newspaper clippings, drawings and my clothes, hung on random hooks around the room and extending into a cute little space that was actually a cupboard under some stairs. I even brought my pet goldfish in its bowl on the bus, all the way from Tickhill via Doncaster to Sheffield.

My landlord, an affable, easygoing Bangladeshi man, would appear every morning and cook breakfast for all 16 students living in the house, plus any blow-ins who may have stayed over. The green mug was the most exciting piece amongst the selection of chipped white crockery in this share house and I quickly claimed it as mine. Surprisingly, no one contested me for it when I moved on, so it came too.

At university, music became more of a passion as I was exposed to new genres – jazz and independent bands, including Caravan, which was one of the less commercial members of the 'prog rock' school and part of the Canterbury music movement. My record player was constantly in use and I would search the second-hand vinyl shops for albums by lesser known artists.

Every cell of my body felt alive with the experiences I was sharing with people from all walks of life, including from different countries – different tastes, different sounds and different substances.

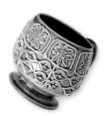

## LOT 67
## THREE CREPE NECK SCARVES, c1920, AND CUTTINGS OF KEITH RICHARDS AND MICK JAGGER
$20–$30

My vibe has been influenced by Keith Richards since long before I was a teenager. At school and university, these pictures graced my walls, and I've had the tattered, fraying 1920s silk neck scarves since the 1970s. For some reason, every time I wear the scarves, 'Keef' comes to mind. Weird huh?

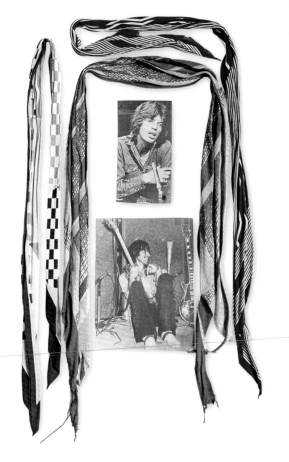

## LOT 68
## FILM SCRIPT FOR *TERMINUS*, WITH PRESS CLIPPINGS, c1975, AND OTHER EPHEMERA
$1–$5

Whilst attending Sheffield University, I spent a lot of time taking part in extra-curricular activities. I wasn't particularly interested in the Students' Union clubs and societies – sports, politics, debates, chess groups and the like – I chose real-life experiences outside the rarefied atmosphere of the campus.

One such experience was working with a new friend, Arthur Ellis, on a short film he'd written, called *Terminus*. This guy was an unemployed crazy genius, constantly and obsessively writing, passionate about his craft and spaghetti westerns – a real artful dodger. His zest for life, sense of adventure, thrill-seeking and challenging of the law knew no bounds.

He would steal food from supermarkets, then walk out openly and stand outside, in the hope of being arrested so he could spend time locked up. He wanted to write with authenticity about life from all angles.

He also never wore socks.

During filming in Sheffield railway station, I was in charge of continuity. Art's unflattering portrayal of the British Rail buffet drew the attention of the authorities and caused a temporary glitch in proceedings. However, this

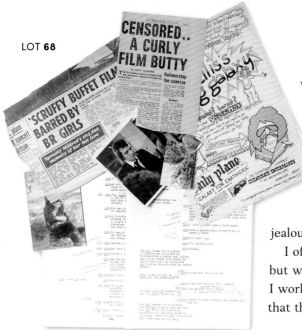

**LOT 68**

was soon resolved, and he lapped up the free press – any publicity was good publicity.

The relationship with my high-school musician boyfriend, Steve Fellows, was becoming messy. For both of us, moving to a different environment in a big city brought new opportunities as well as challenges, and mistrust and jealousies began to tear us apart.

I often felt alone, this time not with sadness, but with excitement and a tantalising trepidation. I worked through my fear by travelling, sensing that the world could be my oyster.

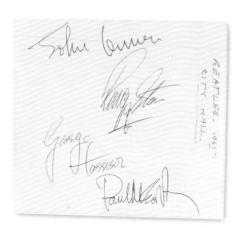

**LOT 69**

## AUTOGRAPHS BY THE BEATLES, c1965, AND PUSSYCAT WILLUM 'AUTOGRAPH', c1960

$7000–$10,000 (WITHDRAWN)

Pussycat Willum was a puppet who appeared with presenters Wally Whyton and Muriel Young on a children's program called *Small Time*.

As a small child, I must have been one of his biggest fans. I wrote in to Rediffusion Television to ask for his autograph and here it is, one of my childhood prize possessions.

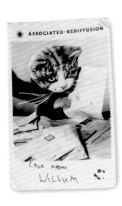

Over the course of filming *Terminus*, I befriended an elderly tea lady, an extra in the film, who had once worked as a cleaner at the Sheffield City Hall. I told her all about my grandmother, Nanny Win, and how we had spent many happy times together going through her old autograph books.

The next day, the lady came up to me and, with a whisper, quietly passed me an envelope containing this page, which she had torn from her own autograph book – a full set of signatures from The Beatles. This became another of my prize possessions.

## LOT 70
### VINTAGE SATIN JACKET, PASSPORT, 1975, AND PHOTOGRAPH, c1980
$20–$30 (WITHDRAWN)

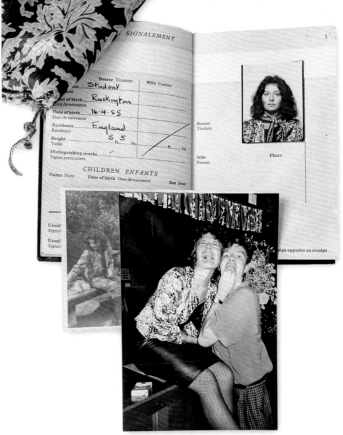

In the mid-1970s, vast areas of Sheffield were incredibly rundown, with empty buildings and outhouses that I loved to explore. One day, on one of my forays, I found a dusty old trunk, clearly untouched for decades, in the corner of a derelict garage. I managed to break it open and inside I discovered a bundle of crumpled garments – filthy, damp, mouldy and stinking. Some of them immediately disintegrated in my hands, others were too tattered to be salvageable, but amongst them, shining in the half light, I could see this beautiful fabric. I pulled it free and was delighted to see that it was a jacket, probably remodelled in the 1940s, and with the potential to live again. I took it home, carefully washed it by hand and patched it where needed. From that day on, with patches on its patches, I have lived in it.

The photographs show me wearing the jacket for my 1975 passport photograph, taken to facilitate a lone trip to Paris, where I stayed for a week or so with some French hippies I had met while they were on exchange at Sheffield University. Whilst in England, one of them had seemed to show an interest in me, even inviting me to Paris. Yet when I arrived, he spent much of his time in bed with another boy, and I returned to Sheffield more confused than ever.

The later photograph, taken in the 1980s, is of me with a friend whose sexual orientation is clear for all to see – so much more comfortable.

I think I will request to be dressed in this jacket when the last breath has left this body.

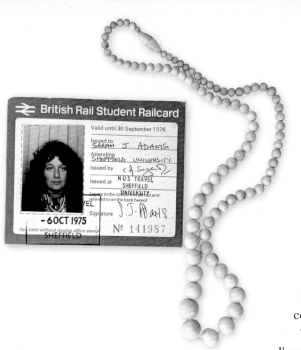

## LOT 71
### IVORY BEAD NECKLACE, c1940, AND BRITISH RAIL STUDENT RAILCARD, 1975
$60–$100

My student railcard was a very important part of my life. I was officially attending Sheffield University, but I was spending most of my time travelling around the country watching bands playing live concerts, or in London.

The graduated bead necklace that I'm wearing in the photograph was a gift from my grandmother.

## LOT 72
### THREE NECKLACES, ONE FROM GREECE, WITH LARGE CERAMIC DECORATIVE BEADS, c1975
$20–$40

During the shooting of *Terminus*, I had planned a trip to Greece for the forthcoming long summer holidays. I travelled on the 'Magic Bus' with three other girls, sitting at the front of the coach as we traversed Europe. It was an adventurous few days involving midnight road accidents, shattered windscreens (with broken glass all over us, and the rest of the journey spent being blown to smithereens in freezing winds), and the filthiest toilet stops I have encountered anywhere in the world. We were all mightily relieved when, after four days, we arrived in Athens.

My relief was short-lived. As we drew into the bus terminus, one of my friends pointed to a solitary young man sitting on the pavement, leaning languidly against the wall. It was the director of the other *Terminus*. He had been aware of our plans, and had hitched from Sheffield to Athens to await my arrival. Talk about travelling to the ends of the earth! I was mortified, flattered, embarrassed and burdened. We spent about a week together, at first dossing down in an empty building (he had already scouted a spot that had 'conveniences'), then moving to beaches on different sides of an island in a vain attempt to "work things out".

Eventually, when things became too painful to bear, he had to leave. I will never forget sitting on the quay, watching him onboard the ferry watching me, as it turned into a black dot on the horizon.

These heavy ceramic beads are my memory of that trip. Their heaviness is nothing compared to the burden of responsibility I feel for that broken man.

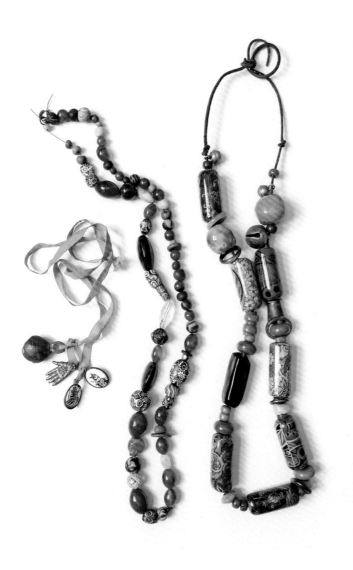

Lot 72

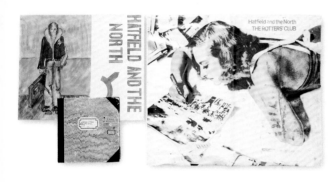

LOT **73**

**HATFIELD AND THE NORTH
VINYL WINDOW STICKER,
AND THE BAND'S ALBUM,
*THE ROTTERS' CLUB*, 1975,
A COMPLETED DIARY, 1975,
AND ONE PAINTING**

$10–$20 (WITHDRAWN)

In the mid-1970s, my musical obsession revolved around a specific band, Hatfield and the North, which was part of a very English underground prog-rock, jazz-impro genre, namely the Canterbury Scene. I was their biggest fan, travelling far and wide to watch them perform, a rare female amongst a sea of duffel-coated fanatical boys.

Gradually, we became friends...

LOT **74**

**PAIR OF SUNGLASSES IN PINK VINYL CASE, c1950,
AND VINTAGE METAL TIN WITH SHAGREEN PAINTED
DECORATION, c1930, CONTAINING A PAIR OF NATIONAL
HEALTH SERVICE (NHS) SUNGLASSES, c1970 (NOT SHOWN)**

$30–$50

In the 1970s, everyone was wearing John Lennon-style round glasses. The NHS specs were a nerdy yet cool version and symbolised to me the band of the same name – National Health – with whom I had become closely affiliated, and which had been formed by members of Hatfield and the North (Lot 73). Mine (seen being worn in the photograph taken in Sheffield in Lot 66), were kept in this little metal tin, painted in a cover of shagreen.

Shagreen is the name given to the skin of a shark or a stingray, which was widely used in the art deco period to decorate small items such as pill boxes, powder compacts and cigarette cases.

Not sure how it happened, but I passed my first-year university exams. A good part of the next two years, whilst I was supposedly attending Sheffield University, were, in fact, spent in London, where I was developing a relationship with Dave Stewart, who had by then left Hatfield and the North and formed National Health, so named after the spectacles he wore.

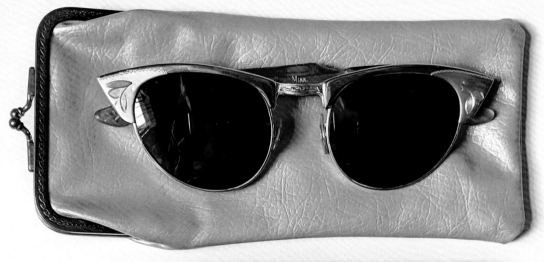

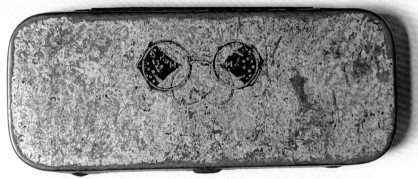

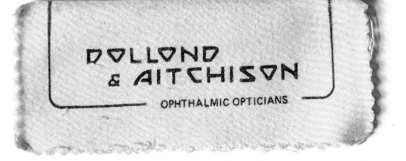

DOLLOND
& AITCHISON

OPHTHALMIC OPTICIANS

LOT **74**

## LOT 75
## HAND-CROCHETED HAT, AN ALBUM AND SINGLE, c1970

$5–$10

Just thought I'd throw in a flying teapot, together with a crochet hat I made, which was a staple part of the new uniform of the time.

Some of you may get the teapot connection, but this link triggers a memory from boarding-school days. We invented paintballing. In our day, it was called Tea Bag Tag. At breakfast time, each table setting would include an industrial-size metal teapot of overly brewed, thick black tea. These teapots contained teabags measuring about four inches (10cm)

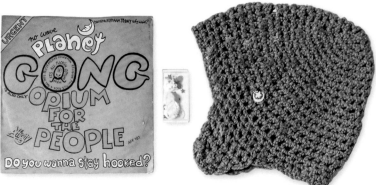

square. We would collect the teabags and at night in the dormitories would get naked, scrambling over and under beds, shrieking and laughing as we lobbed cold, wet teabags at each other. It was hilarious fun, and the winner was the one with the fewest brown 'hits' on their bare flesh.

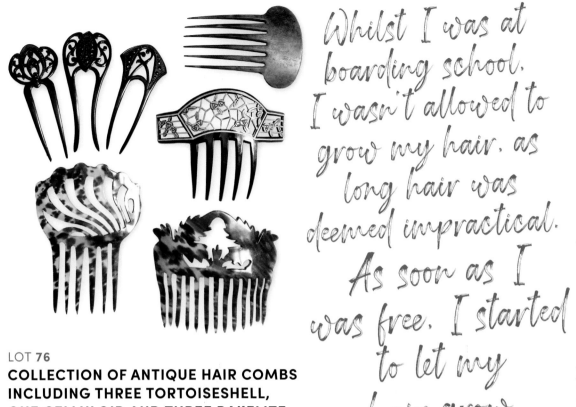

*Whilst I was at boarding school, I wasn't allowed to grow my hair, as long hair was deemed impractical. As soon as I was free, I started to let my hair grow.*

## LOT 76

**COLLECTION OF ANTIQUE HAIR COMBS INCLUDING THREE TORTOISESHELL, ONE CELLULOID AND THREE BAKELITE**

$150–$200

The art nouveau celluloid and Bakelite combs were made in Europe and date from the early 1900s, one features Chinoiserie decoration. The tortoiseshell combs were made later and originate from the Pacific Islands.

I used these combs regularly when I was in my 20s. Whilst I was at boarding school, I wasn't allowed to grow my hair, as long hair was deemed impractical. As soon as I was free, I started to let my hair grow. I was inspired by the hairdos of the women of the early 1900s, the 'Gibson Girls', who wore big upsweeps of long, thick hair, as seen in the enamel brooch that forms part of the collection offered in Lot 52. In 1970s England, it was hard to find interesting, dependable hair accessories capable of holding up a thick head of hair, and these traditional combs, bought in jumble sales in Sheffield and London, were both practical and individual. They all had previously belonged to someone else, which, for me, was a contributing attraction – a link to another life.

## COLLECTION OF PLASTIC HAIR CLIPS, 1970s AND 1980s, AND THREE PHOTOGRAPHS

$5–$10

The photos show me in the late 1970s and 80s in Chiswick and Bermondsey markets. I still wear my bag slung across my body, an Indian cotton scarf, the colour orange and these plastic hair clips.

LOT **78**

## BOUND COPY OF THESIS, *REGIONAL IMAGERY IN ENGLAND: NORTHERNERS AND SOUTHERNERS,* 1976 (NOT SHOWN)

$5–$10

By the time I reached university, I had been exposed to, been guilty of, and been the victim of social stereotyping. I decided to make it the topic of the thesis that was a part of my final assessment for a Bachelor of Arts in Sociology.

My parents had received a bursary to assist in paying for my enrolment at an all-girls private school in the Home Counties. As the daughter of a lowly RAF officer, I was alienated from most of the other girls, many of whom were daughters of (multi) millionaires, (huge) landowners in places as far afield as Australia, and (mega) businessmen with offshore ventures in places such as Jersey.

At 16, I had rebelled and requested to attend a comprehensive school in Yorkshire, where I was quite clearly a foreigner. I spoke differently, lived in a new house in a posh village, had lived abroad and had only attended private schools. I may as well have landed from Mars.

Although I had achieved good results in my 'O' and 'A' levels, I never considered myself an academic, so felt something of a fraud (imposter syndrome) at being at university. I couldn't wait to complete my formal education, as I naively felt this meant I had fulfilled other people's expectations of me. At least I had fulfilled the ones they had paid for, which gave me an enormous sense of freedom.

The day after I finished my final university exams, I moved from Sheffield to London, where I would spend four years living in a basement flat near Strand-on-the-Green, Chiswick, with my new keyboard-playing boyfriend,

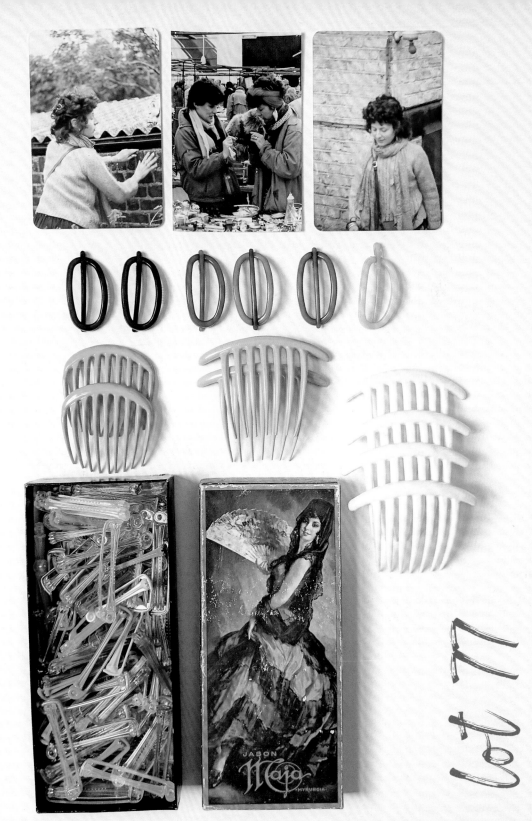

Lot 77

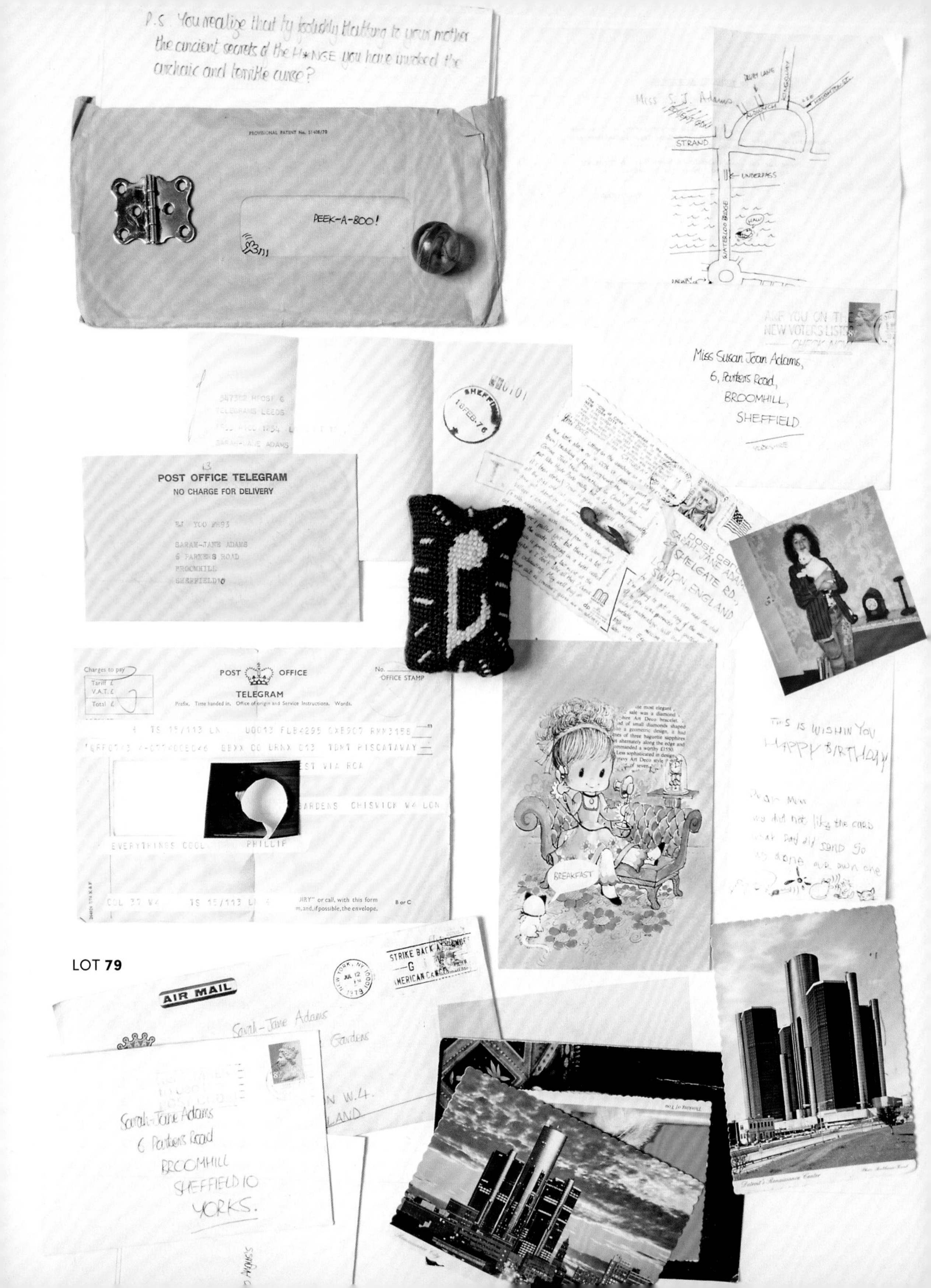
P.S. You realize that by foolishly blabbing to your mother the ancient secrets of the H*NGE you have invoked the archaic and terrible curse?
PEEK-A-BOO!
Miss S. J. Adams
STRAND
UNDERPASS
WATERLOO BRIDGE
ARE YOU ON THE NEW VOTERS LISTS? CHECK NOW
Miss Susan Joan Adams,
6, Parkers Road,
BROOMHILL,
SHEFFIELD
POST OFFICE TELEGRAM
NO CHARGE FOR DELIVERY
SARAH-JANE ADAMS
6 PARKERS ROAD
BROOMHILL
SHEFFIELD 10
18 FEB 76
POST OFFICE
TELEGRAM
EVERYTHINGS COOL
PHILLIP
BREAKFAST
THIS IS WISHIN YOU
HAPPY BIRTHDAY
AIR MAIL
STRIKE BACK
Sarah-Jane Adams
Sarah-Jane Adams
6 Parkers Road
BROOMHILL
SHEFFIELD 10
YORKS.
Detroit's Renaissance Center

LOT **79**

Dave Stewart. His flatmate at the time, a hippie who had a business building giant PA systems in an arch under Kew Bridge, very kindly drove his truck between Sheffield and London to assist me in the big move.

I was taking ownership of my life and now was solely responsible for myself and decisions about my future.

## LOT 79

### SELECTED EPHEMERA, 1976–1979, INCLUDING A HANDMADE PIN CUSHION DEPICTING A SHINING QUAVER, AND HINGE BROOCH

$10–$20 (WITHDRAWN)

This collection is a small part of the ephemera I have kept from the times when I was commuting between Sheffield and London. I was living de facto with the de facto leader of the band.

The letters, postcards, writings and sketches are from Dave, some from when he was touring in the USA. He also made the hinge brooch, seen top left, from a PA flight-case hinge.

His immaculate handwriting reads: "PS. You realise that by foolishly blabbing to your mother the ancient secrets of the H*NGE you have invoked the archaic and terrible curse?" Humour and the understanding of symbolism are always an attractive characteristic.

The customised pink card he made is particularly charming to me.

*I was living de facto with the de facto leader of the band.*

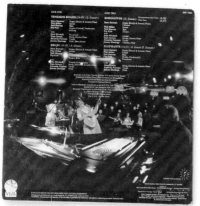

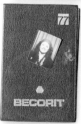

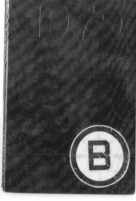

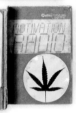

## LOT 80

### ALBUM COVER BY NATIONAL HEALTH, 1978, AND THREE DIARIES, LATE 1970s

$10–$20 (WITHDRAWN)

The front cover of National Health's first album shows an image of the band shot ironically inside a National Health hospital. The back cover was shot in Ronnie Scott's jazz club in Frith Street, Soho. Ronnie Scott, the legendary jazz musician, is playing the piano and, in another nod to the National Health, I'm dressed as a nurse, pretending to play band member Neil Murray's bass guitar.

I documented my life with Dave Stewart and my time with the band in these, and many other diaries.

## LOT 81

### VINTAGE BLACK METAL CASH TIN, c1940, CONTAINING MINIATURE ENAMEL PAINTS AND VARIOUS ITEMS, INCLUDING HANDMADE WOODEN LIQUORICE ALLSORTS, c1970

$30–$40

In the 1970s, I sewed, wove macramé wall hangings, plant holders and lampshades, created leather guitar straps and other small items, and generally enjoyed all kinds of craftwork. This love of crafting developed into jewellery making.

Soon, every other medium was cast aside as I focused on learning new techniques, designing different items of jewellery. An earlier obsession with the minutiae of stationery was readily transferred to the minutiae of jewellery and here, in a tiny way, a business was born. I briefly attended silversmithing classes, but my hands shook too much, so that didn't last long. (See the silver quaver brooch in Lot 79.)

Living in Chiswick meant that, as well as sourcing odds and ends in the local jumble sales, I could also nip up on the number 27 bus to Wardour Street, in London's West End, where an old-school store, J. Blundell & Sons (established in 1839) supplied jewellery findings, silver wire and all the other components required by the jewellery trade. I was in heaven. I made earrings using antique beads, miniature components from modelling sets and feathers. I also created handmade oddities such as the wooden liquorice allsorts sweeties shown here.

There was a little shop in a laneway off Turnham Green, near Chiswick, which took items on consignment and not only provided me with a small income, but also an awareness that I had found my forte in the world of jewellery. I developed a great thirst for knowledge and exploration, finding ways to combine creativity with enquiry to create a niche where I could be as comfortable and as challenged as I felt fit.

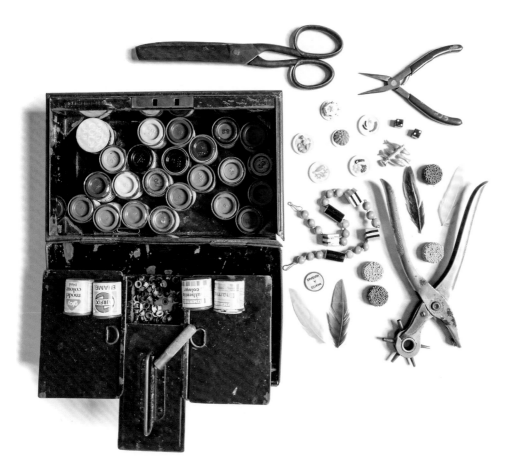

## QUEEN ELIZABETH II SILVER JUBILEE COMMEMORATION CROWN, 1977, AND GOLDEN VIRGINIA TOBACCO TIN WITH VARIOUS EPHEMERA, PHOTOGRAPH AND SECURITY PASS

$5–$10

The photograph shows me backstage after a National Health gig, exhausted but happy. Cross-referencing with my diaries, the security pass, dated 6 February 1976, indicates that the gig was at Trent Polytechnic. At that time, I was living, breathing and working with the band. At home, I was the gofer, secretary, phone-answerer and all-round assistant and listener. On the road, I toured with the band as the lighting person, often travelling

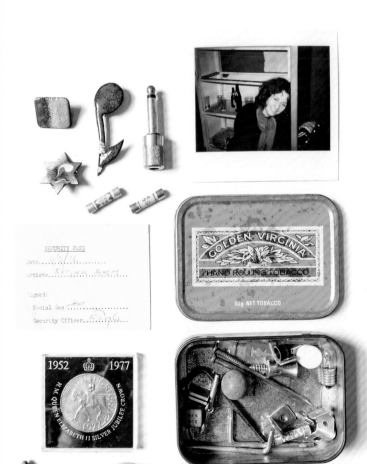

ahead in the truck with the roadies. I was responsible for hiring, setting up and working the lights at each venue. This frequently involved discussions and negotiations with the event's in-house workers, who, without exception, were always male. Funnily enough, I never thought this was strange; I was simply one of the boys and enjoyed the camaraderie of working in a man's world.

This tobacco tin contains my spares: a jack plug, fuses, knobs, amp corner protectors and bulbs for amps, along with a few examples of my first attempts at jewellery-making in the form of enamel badges. The red shining quaver is particularly special to me, as a shining quaver became the 'logo' for Dave Stewart.

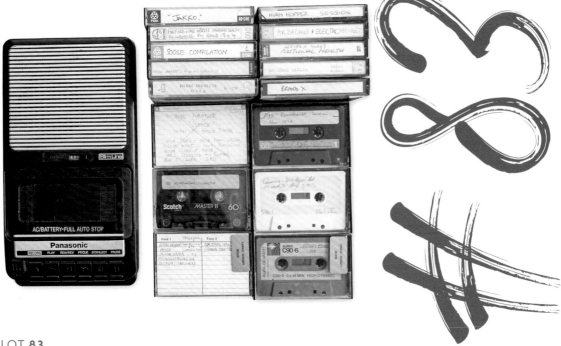

LOT **83**

## SLIMLINE PANASONIC TAPE RECORDER AND VARIOUS
## USED CASSETTE TAPES, c1975

$80–$120

My partner, Dave Stewart, was a classically trained musician who wrote
complicated multi-instrumental scores for the band. Publishing and royalty
cheques were few and far between. We spent many an afternoon loitering
in Vernon Yard off Portobello Road (where Virgin Records had their
offices), hoping for an advance. My babysitting work and jewellery
creations provided minimal income, and we often lived hand-to-mouth.

Many successful bands in those days couldn't play their instruments, let
alone chart the scores required for publishing royalties to be collected.
So, periodically, we would receive from Virgin pre-release copies of albums,
so that the musician in the house could create a 'lead sheet' (a musical
notation of the melody, lyrics and harmony of songs). The album would be
recorded onto a cassette tape, which was then played, stop-start, stop-start,
stop-start, in this Panasonic tape recorder, so that the lead line could be
found (sometimes with difficulty), transcribed and returned to the Virgin
Publishing legal department.

This process could take weeks to complete, depending on the complexity
of the music and the intelligibility of the lyrics. For this, Dave received the
princely sum of 50 quid per album.

We had many albums, pre-release copies of all genres, from punk to rock to 'tragic'. One Sunday, to earn some cash, I took a load of stuff up to the flea market at Camden Lock and set up shop on the cobblestones outside Dingwalls. I was selling clothes and paraphernalia, and had a box of albums going for £1 each on the ground at the front.

This was the day I probably made the biggest blunder of my working life. In the box was a pre-release copy of Mike Oldfield's *Tubular Bells*. This album launched Virgin Records and was the third-best-selling album in the UK in the 1970s. I watched two boys flicking through the box, pulling that one out. They asked the price. "One pound," I chirped. As they inspected the label, they gasped when they saw it was a pre-release copy. The price had been stated and, always a woman of my word, I let it go, already aware of my mistake.

I haven't researched what this item would be worth today, but at least we had food on the table that night.

## LOT 84

## COLLECTION OF BOOKS, HANDWRITTEN PAPERS, STOCK INVENTORIES AND SALES LISTS, AUTUMN 1978

$5–$10

This collection shows in meticulous detail the absolute beginnings of my business. It was 18 September 1978, a Monday – the day of the flea market in Old Covent Garden Market.

Self-employment came to me through necessity as well as choice. I was living with a musician, the scribe of these papers, in a basement flat in Chiswick. Earnings from both our endeavours were sporadic and lean. One day, in the autumn of 1978, I had to make the decision whether to spend our last 20 pence on toothpaste or potatoes.

Realising the situation was dire, I looked around the flat: I had collected an array of interesting bits and pieces; I was a great fan of jumble sales and thrift stores; I had an eye for the odd and the unusual; and I would travel miles on my bicycle to local church halls and community centres, where charities sold people's donated cast-offs.

I figured that if I found this stuff interesting, perhaps others might, too. But how to find these people? I bought *The Evening Standard*, a London-wide newspaper, and scoured the trade section.

Eureka! I spotted a small advert: "Stallholders wanted for the New Jubilee Market, opening on the site of the old Covent Garden market."

The wholesale fruit and vegetable market, which for centuries had been housed in Covent Garden, had, in 1974, moved to Vauxhall. Restoration works on the old site were now complete and it was time to open the new-look Covent Garden, offering different daily attractions. I became one of the inaugural 'antiques' dealers at the Monday market, and my business was launched.

I never had to choose between toothpaste and potatoes again.

---

### Soose's Business — MONTH 1
25·8·78 — 9·10·78

**Expenditure.**

| Date | £ | (Page) | |
|---|---|---|---|
| 25/8/78 – 9/8/78 | 46·55 | (1) | |
| 9/9/78 – 17/9/78 | 50·18 | (2) | |
| 17/9/78 – 20/9/78 | 29·05 | (3) | 2ND. WEEK |
| 20/9/78 – 23/9/78 | 28·70 | (4) | |
| 24/9/78 – 8/10/78 (incl. STALL for 13 WEEKS) | 131·90 | (5) | 3RD. + 4TH. WEEKS |
| 8/10/78 | 36·77 | (6) | 4TH. WEEK |
| 8/10/78 (contd.) | 21·85 | (7) | |
| **£345·00** | TOTAL (25/8/78 – 8/10/78.) | | |

**Income**

| | £ | |
|---|---|---|
| COVENT GARDEN 18/9/78 | 76·05 | 1ST. WEEK |
| COVENT GARDEN 25/9/78 | 56·65 | 2ND. WEEK |
| COVENT GARDEN 2/10/78 | 30·70 | 3RD. WEEK |
| PORTOBELLO RD. 7/10/78 | 33·30 | 4TH. WEEK |
| COVENT GARDEN 9/10/78 | 59·40 | |
| * **£256·10** | TOTAL (18/9/78 – 9/10/78) | |

* Loss of £88·90 on 1st month; but £50 of this buys stall for 13 weeks, + some of rest (i.e. leather bag) is to start business.

---

**Income**

| | | £ |
|---|---|---|
| PORTOBELLO RD. | 11/11/78 | 49·00 |
| COV. GDN. | 13/11/78 | 78·00 |
| PORTOBELLO RD. | 18/11/78 | 91·75 |
| CAMDEN | 19/11/78 | 29·00 |
| COV. GDN. | 20/11/78 | 71·50 |
| PORTOBELLO RD. | 23/11/78 | 79·75 |
| CAMDEN | 26/11/78 | 29·70 |
| COV. GDN. | 27/11/78 | 91·75 |
| PORTOBELLO RD. | 30/11/78 | 44·00 |
| CAMDEN | 3/12/78 | 82·43 |
| COV. GDN. | 4/12/78 | 59·25 |
| PORTOBELLO RD. | 8/12/78 | 14·00 |
| " | 9/12/78 | 81·50 |
| CAMDEN | 10/12/78 | 46·95 |
| | | **£848·58** TOTAL (10/11/78 – 10/12/78) |

Profit of £286·40 on Month 3.

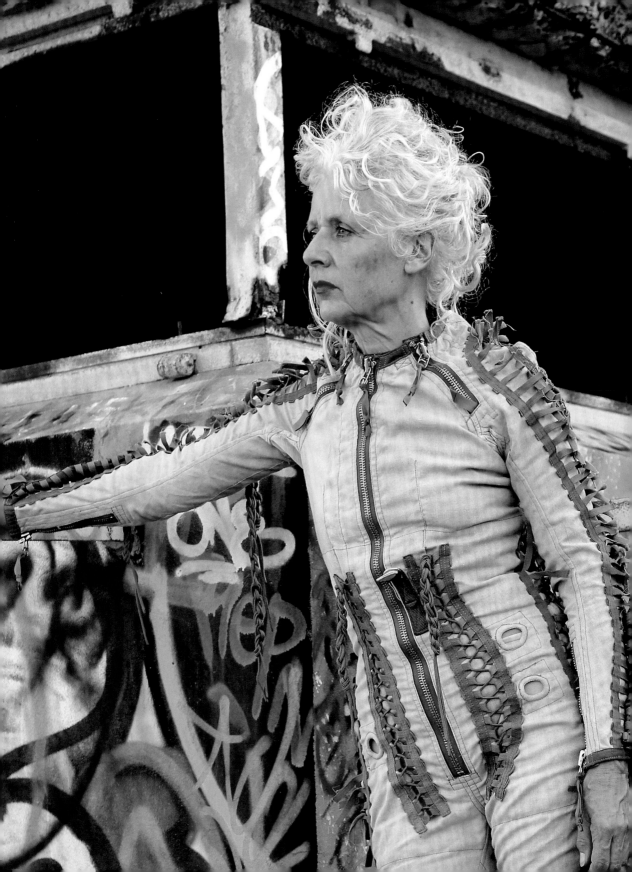

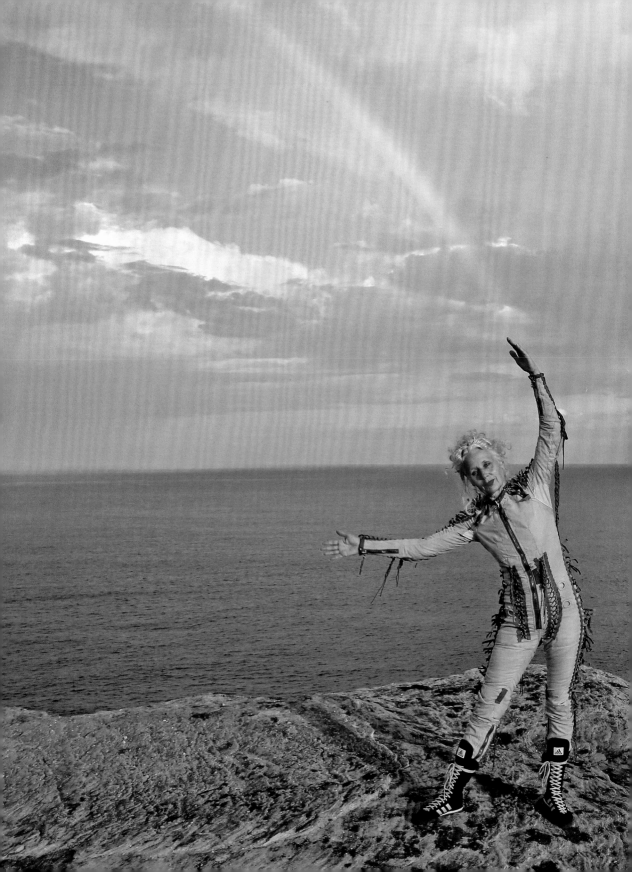

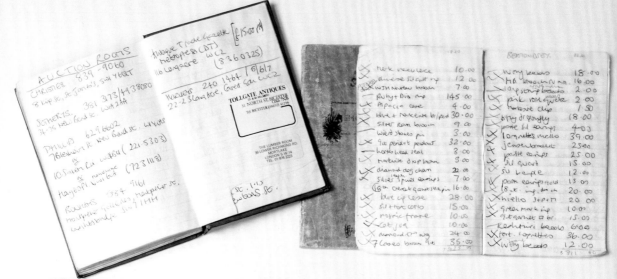

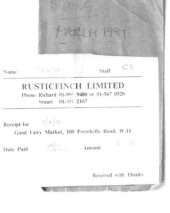

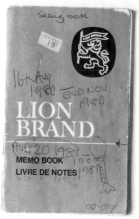

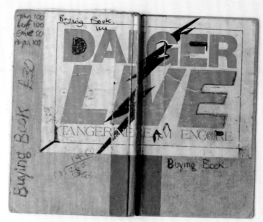

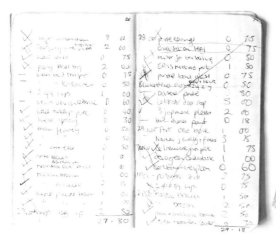

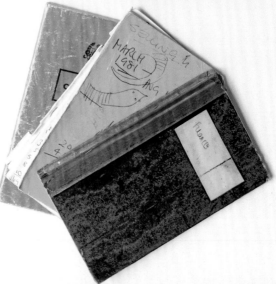

LOT **84**

# living off our wits

## LOT 85

## COLLECTION OF 10 VINTAGE NOVELTY EGG CUPS, WITH REFERENCE BOOK, PHOTOGRAPH, c1979, AND MAGAZINE ARTICLE, DATED 1992

$350–$500 (MORE EGG CUPS AVAILABLE ON REQUEST)

I had come to realise that one (wo)man's trash is another (wo)man's treasure. At this stage, I was scouring antiques shops as well as jumble sales and markets. I plucked up the courage to enter establishments of all levels. By mainstream society's standards, I looked like "something the cat had dragged in", so I needed an excuse that would open doors to such places, to create an opportunity to strike up a conversation. Thus, I began my collection of novelty egg cups. I would enter all antique and jewellery stores, asking the seemingly innocent question, "Do you have any novelty egg cups for sale?" You'd be surprised how many people did.

Once the ice had been broken, regardless of whether an egg cup or two were purchased, I would ask the proprietors questions about their stock. I was a sponge, soaking up knowledge, always researching, coming to understand how objects reflect what is happening in the world and seeing the association between the different disciplines of architecture, literature, cultural artefacts, jewellery and clothing. My brain was in overload and I was in heaven.

The most interesting egg cup shown here is the World War II goose-stepping goose wearing a German helmet at the top of this collection. A clever play on words – as in "don't be a goose" – it implies that Nazism is for someone who is 'a goose'. Also shown is a Charlie Chaplin caricature, along with various generic lustreware birds.

Years later, in Sydney, a large part of my collection was featured in the Easter edition of *Good Weekend* magazine and subsequently sold in the former Mosman Antique Centre.

The photograph shows me in the Good Fairy Market, Portobello Road. On my stall in the background, can be seen the odd egg cup. I'm also wearing the scarf referred to in Lot 115, 'Memoirs of a Greek scarf'.

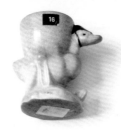

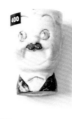

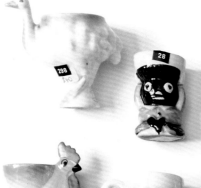

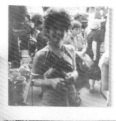

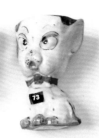

## COLLECTING
# EGG CUPS
### AN INTRODUCTION TO POCILLOVY
### by WINNIE FREEMAN

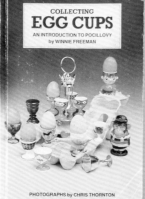

PHOTOGRAPHS by CHRIS THORNTON

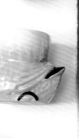

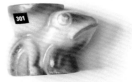

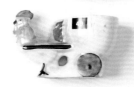

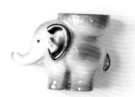

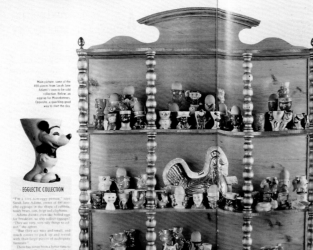

# BEST WEEKEND
## Stand and deliver

DESIGN

### EGGLECTIC COLLECTION

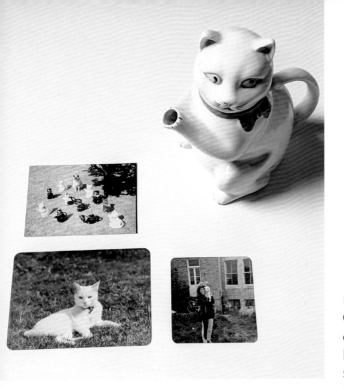

LOT **86**

**CERAMIC WHITE CAT TEAPOT, c1930, AND THREE PHOTOGRAPHS, LATE 1970s**

$250–$300

Ronnie and Reggie, the two kittens who lived with us in our basement flat, were named after the Kray twins, notorious criminals who through their gang, The Firm, ran East London's underworld during the 1950s and 60s. During my early days as an antiques dealer in the late 1970s, I had built a collection of art deco teapots in the shape of cats, seen here in one of these photographs. I subsequently sold the collection, but held onto this rare one. I valued it more, as it reminded me of my twin kittens, little Ronnie and Reggie.

In the photo I am wearing my pride and joy – my first and probably only 'serious' clothing purchase – a black leather jacket, referred to in Lot 51. It cost me fifty quid, a small fortune, but I lived in that jacket. On cold, wet winter mornings, I would stand at my corner pitch at Covent Garden market, my feet deep in a puddle. Dressed in this jacket, with my leather pants tucked into gumboots customised with studded leather spurs and lined with newspaper for warmth, I felt hot, invincible and totally in my element. I was amongst the real people, the hustlers, banding together against the elements and living off our wits.

The bag slung over my shoulder contained all my stock, all my worldly possessions and my livelihood – antique jewellery to sell at the markets. I was well on my way – my business was growing, I was free-spirited and brave, and my world was there for the making.

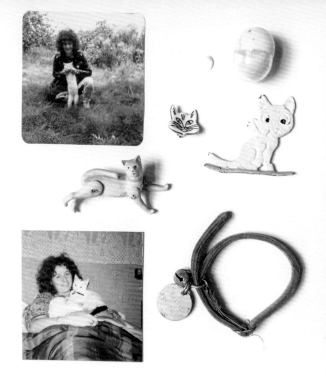

*a sense of happiness, expansion and fulfilment*

## LOT **87**

### HANDPAINTED VICTORIAN BISQUE ARTICULATED WHITE CAT TOY, LATE 1800s, LEAD-PAINTED WHITE CAT, 1920s, AND VARIOUS EPHEMERA

$300–$400

In the late 1970s, I was drawn to the superstition around our two cats – the belief that they bring good luck and calm, and can enhance the psychic power of their companion. Certainly, during the time that I spent sharing my life with Ronnie and Reggie, I began to understand a sense of happiness, expansion and fulfilment. The plastic container shown holds some fur and a small white tooth, and with the green velvet collar, they are direct connections to my furry friends.

The small articulated cat was probably a toy from a doll's house.

The phone number engraved on the metal collar tag is imprinted in my memory. Our phone never stopped ringing, as pretty much everything concerning the band was organised from our flat. Gigs, rehearsals, jam sessions, equipment, van hire, interviews, work bills and payments – they all came through this phone number. Whenever the phone rang, I didn't know who to expect at the other end, so I always answered, "Nine, nine, five, five, double-0, five."

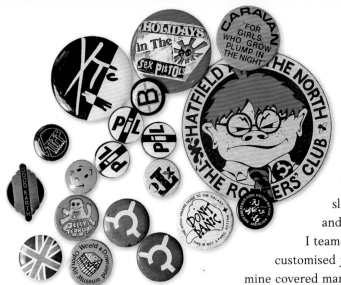

LOT **88**

## COLLECTION OF PINS AND BADGES, 1970s

$30–$50

These decorated the lapels or rolled-up sleeves of my vintage 1930s maroon and blue striped school blazer, which I teamed with a patched pair of threadbare customised jeans. Badges indicate allegiances and mine covered many groups as I developed a sense of self that was difficult to contain or compartmentalise. In a moment of clarity, my father had commented that blue jeans are merely another uniform, another indication of allegiance. I have never worn 'uncustomised' blue jeans. The mainly music-industry pins include those of the bands Caravan, Hatfield and the North, XTC, Public Image Ltd, Sex Pistols and Bruford – along with Good Earth, a recording studio owned by legendary producer Tony Visconti, and *The Hitchhiker's Guide to the Galaxy*.

LOT **89**

## COPY OF PUBLIC IMAGE LTD DEBUT ALBUM, *FIRST ISSUE*, 1978, AND VARIOUS CONCERT TICKETS

$10–$20

One of the last events I attended during my time in the music scene was the 1978 concert in Paris by the recently formed Public Image Ltd (PIL). As part of the Virgin Records contingent, a bunch of us were invited to go to France and support Johnny Rotten's new band. The gig was a complete shambles and sadly impressed very few people, I suspect Johnny Rotten included, as he spent most of the time with his back to the audience or off stage. The performance was halted several times as people gobbed and chucked bottles – and pretty much anything – at the band. The sound was appalling and the light show (which I'd been keen to see, in my own role as a band lighting person) non-existent.

The concert tickets pictured are: Public Image Ltd, 1978; Rolling Stones, 2003 (twice); Eminem, 2011 and 2019; Paolo Nutini, 2009; Prince, 2012; 5SOS, 2014; Red Hot Chili Peppers, 2019. I attended most of them alone.

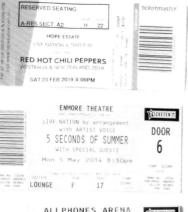

RESERVED SEATING
A-RES SECT A2    ROW H    SEAT 22    COMP $0.00

ticketmaster

HOPE ESTATE
LIVE NATION & TRIPLE M

RED HOT CHILI PEPPERS
AUSTRALIA & NEW ZEALAND 2019

SAT 23 FEB 2019 4:00PM

CONDITIONS OF ENTRY

---

ENMORE THEATRE

TICKETEK

LIVE NATION by arrangement
with ARTIST VOICE

5 SECONDS OF SUMMER
WITH SPECIAL GUESTS

Mon 5 May 2014 8:30pm

DOOR
6

SECTION LOUNGE    ROW F    SEAT 17

---

ALLPHONES ARENA
AT SYDNEY OLYMPIC PARK

TICKETEK

VAN EGMOND GROUP, CHUGG ENTERTAINMENT,
MAX & CHANNEL [V] PRESENT

PRINCE
WELCOME 2 AUSTRALIA 2012

Sat 12 May 2012 8:00pm

MAIN
CONCOURSE

DOOR
7

7    7    JJ    141

---

RECEIPT - NOT VALID FOR ENTRY
ENMORE THEATRE

TICKETEK

PAOLO NUTINI - Fri 30 Oct 2009 8:00pm
MS SARAH-JANE ADAMS
#86099596(tel)

---

SYDNEY FOOTBALL STADIUM

EMINEM
TOUR YOURSELF
WITH SPECIAL GUESTS

Gates Open 4:00pm

PARK KD ENTRY

384Y57    R    67

---

ROLLING STONES

TICKETEK

---

DOOR
3

ROLLING STONES
ENMORE THEATRE
A Non-Smoking Venue

LICKS WORLD TOUR 2003
STRICTLY NO CAMERAS OR RECORDING DEVICES

Tue 18 Feb 2003 7:30pm

SEATED BEHIND STANDING DANCEFLOOR

SECTION STALLS    ROW L    SEAT 12    $56.05

NM018FEB2003PC

---

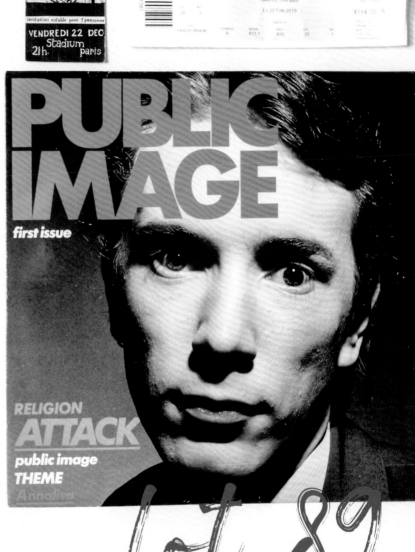

concert

public image ltd.

invitation valable pour 1 personne

VENDREDI 22 DEC
21h. Stadium paris

---

ANZ STADIUM
NO CAMERAS OR AUDIO/VISUAL RECORDING DEVICES ALLOWED

TICKETEK

EMINEM
RAPTURE 2019
A TEG DAINTY PRESENTATION

Fri 22 Feb 2019

GATE A

$114.70

---

PUBLIC IMAGE

first issue

RELIGION
ATTACK
public image
THEME
Annalisa

lot 89

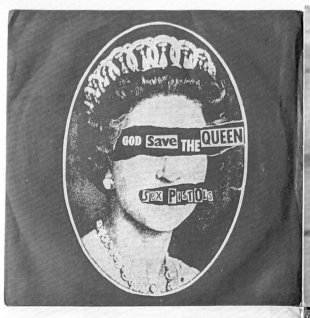

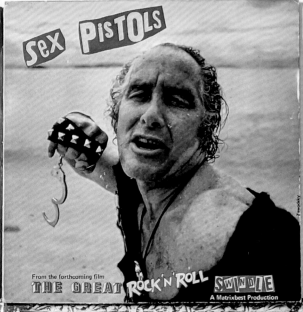

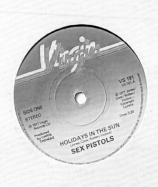

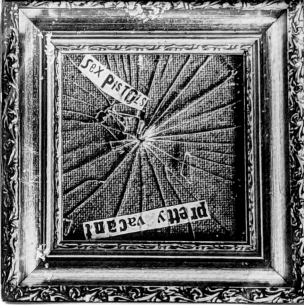

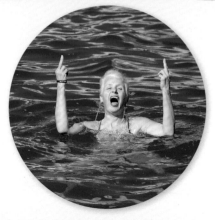

LOT **90**

## LOT **90**

## FOUR 45RPM SINGLES BY THE SEX PISTOLS

$250–$350

The singles are 'God Save the Queen', 'Pretty Vacant', 'Holidays in the Sun', all released in 1977, and 'The Great Rock 'n' Roll Swindle', featuring Ronnie Biggs, released in 1979.

London, how I loved you. To me, your name signifies wildness and boldness, and living in your heart meant those characteristics became a part of me. The sense of being home, possibly for the first time in my life, gave me strength to discover who I truly was and to evolve into who I wanted to be. Times changed, trends came and went, and I found myself straddled across many subcultures. The time came when I knew I had to move on from the once-eclectic scene in Chiswick, one that now had become too familiar. So, I moved into a room in a squat in Battersea.

## LOT **91**

## SILVER BROOCH WITH EMERALD AND RUBY SETTING, BOXED, DATE AND ORIGIN UNKNOWN

$500–$600 (WITHDRAWN)

During the late 1970s, I served my apprenticeship by immersing myself in the street markets of London. A favourite haunt was Whitechapel (the brown collection on the Monopoly board) in the East End, specifically the pre-dawn Brick Lane Sunday flea market.

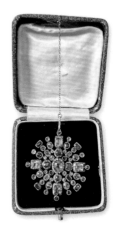

Brick Lane traditionally has been a haven for immigrants seeking a new life away from persecution in their homelands. The demographic was changing again, as the established Jewish and Irish communities were being joined by Bangladeshi families. I remember them, the women wearing exotically garish polyester saris under mismatched nylon cardigans, the men clad in traditional white cotton kurtas and pyjamas, their clothes incongruous under the shapeless overcoats and heavy black boots protecting them against London's inclement climate.

In those days, we would fossick by torchlight amongst the barrows in the back streets and, when the sun came up, we would go to the local bagel bakery for breakfast. Heirlooms from other lives and foreign lands became my obsession, my escape, my livelihood and my new reality.

As soon as I set eyes on this piece, I recognised the gems in this brooch, yet to this day, am not able to ascertain its background. Could it be very early English, Austro-Hungarian, French or even Indian in origin? The mystery of this treasure captivates me and until I have unravelled its secrets, I am not yet ready to move it on. My calling in life – my trade – is to act as a conduit for special, pre-loved items of jewellery to now find their places. Presently, the place for this piece is with me.

## LOT 92
## COLLECTION OF 'LUCKY BLACK CATS', INCLUDING A VICTORIAN LEAD PIN CUSHION
$150–$200

Life in the markets exposed me to many and varied items. While it could have been overwhelming, by putting my money where my mouth was and supporting myself by living the daily hustle, I was developing the skill of selectivity, appreciating what was desirable and understanding a sensible way to present and on-sell. It quickly became apparent to me that collections were generally more desirable than random single pieces. Everyone loves a story, and the traders I supplied loved being able to present one.

I only had my foot on the bottom rung of the ladder, but I was hungry and had found my passion; I never once questioned that I was in the wrong profession. Every day was an adventure. I would build collections of items, stockpiling and releasing when the time was right. I was now living in one small room in a Battersea squat, having left my boyfriend and the tranquillity of Chiswick, so those collections had to be small and easily stashable, as there was little security in the house.

As well as learning about gems and jewellery, I was learning about 'objects of virtue' – small, beautifully made curiosities and collectibles, such as enamels, engravings, boxes and trinkets. The sale of one such

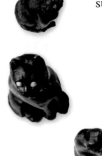
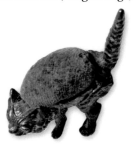
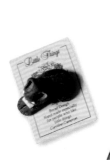

collection – ceramic half-dolls, or pin-cushion dolls – would later provide the deposit on my first house.

Sometimes I would hold back extremely small and cute items, such as the tiny cats shown here, to form the basis of a new collection. You can't really go wrong with a lucky black cat or two.

## LOT 93
## 15CT GOLD MUSICAL STAVE BROOCH, STONES MISSING, BOXED, c1900
$400–$500

This little brooch is a secret token of love. The stave of music with the treble clef is followed by the notes D, E and A, followed by 'REST', spelling 'DEAREST'.

In the late 1970s and early 80s, every Saturday I could be found at my stall in the now, long-gone 'Good Fairy Market'. In those days many celebrities could be seen walking around the markets; even Princess Margaret would wander through, 'undercover' in a headscarf and sunglasses. One time, my high-school sweetheart, Stephen Fellows (by now the lead guitarist and singer in the Comsat Angels) came by, as he had heard that I was '*selling antiques on market day*'. He subsequently penned a song, 'Forever Young', which was released in 1985.

One Saturday I was behind my stall, dressed in my father's RAF flying overalls (which, incidentally I still wear), with this little brooch pinned just above the RAF 'wings'. I looked up, straight into the blue eyes of Mick Jagger, who I could tell had noticed the musical brooch I was wearing. Jerry Hall was right behind him, and I delighted in watching them amble off together, knowing that I had just had a secret 'moment' with Mick Jagger!

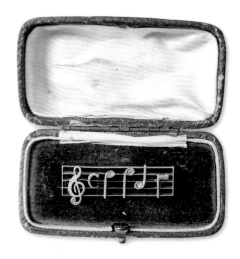

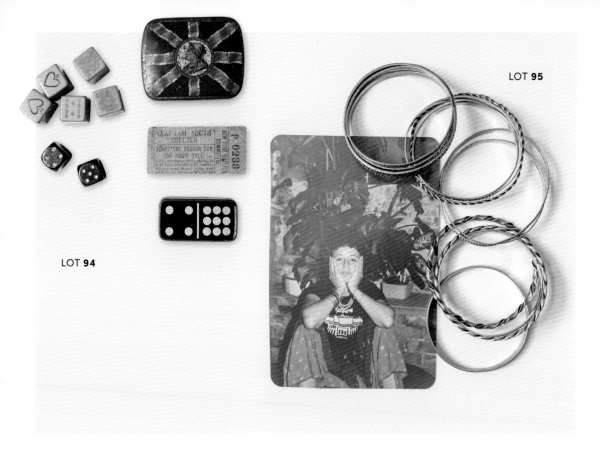

LOT **95**

LOT **94**

## LOT **94**

### TIN DEPICTING QUEEN VICTORIA, c1880,
### CONTAINING A SET OF POKER DICE, c1950,
### A 'DOMINO' TIN, c1900, AND TICKET

$60–$100

I started to make enough money to feel confident enough to pay rent, so, in the early 1980s, I moved into a share flat in Clapham Junction.

This interesting collection of random objects tells a little bit about life in Clapham during wartime and earlier. During World War II, a number of London Underground stations were used as shelters from the German air raids devastating the city during the Blitz. The ticket shown here was for one night's accommodation at the Clapham South shelter. Thousands of people would gather underground, where a thriving community existed and where folks continued to be housed long after the end of the war.

## LOT 95

### COLLECTION OF SILVER BANGLES, AND PHOTOGRAPH, 1980

$50–$60

The photograph shows I'm already in my comfortable place gathering a good bangle stack, wearing a wrist full of silver bangles. Other than the odd piece of fabric or string, bangles are the only form of bracelet I wear, for many reasons. Initially, it was comfort and safety, as bangles don't slip off easily, don't have clasps to catch on things and can't come undone. As I continued to wear my silver bangles, their tinkling sound comforted me and encouraged me to go out into the world and be, live, experience.

A silver or gold full-circle bangle is believed to capture and contain energy, which is absorbed into the body. The positioning of a bangle in contact with the pulse is believed to encourage good blood circulation.

The Uptown Theatre T-shirt I am wearing was a gift from my muso ex-boyfriend, Dave Stewart, who had recently returned to London from a US tour with Bruford.

## LOT 96

### ONE LEATHER BOOKMARK, c1965, AND FIVE BOOKS: *RUBAIYAT OF OMAR KHAYYAM*, 1971 EDITION; *FULL TILT*, DERVLA MURPHY, 1965; *THE THIRD EYE*, LOBSANG RAMPA, 1956; *A SHORT WALK IN THE HINDU KUSH*, ERIC NEWBY, 1958; AND *THE FOURTH WAY*, PD OUSPENSKY, 1971

$10–$15

The leather bookmark was a childhood treasure. By now, I was reading copious travel books. My horizons were widening, and I knew it would not be long before I would be exploring further.

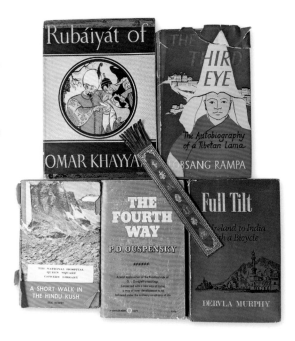

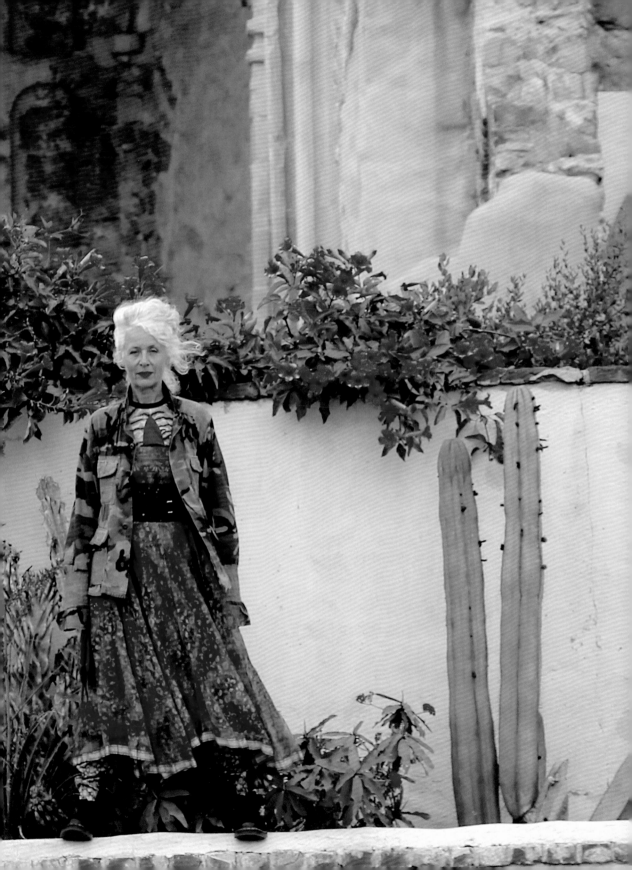

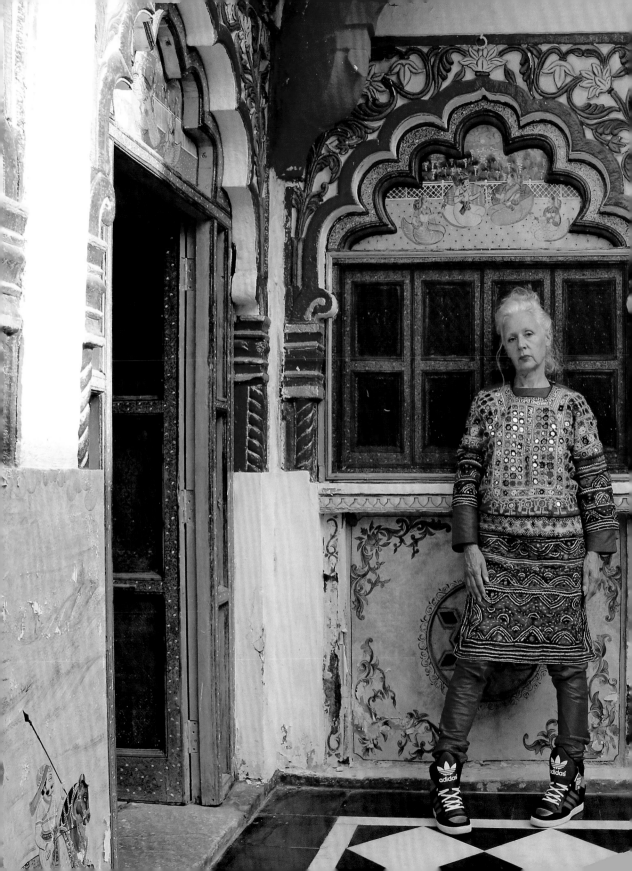

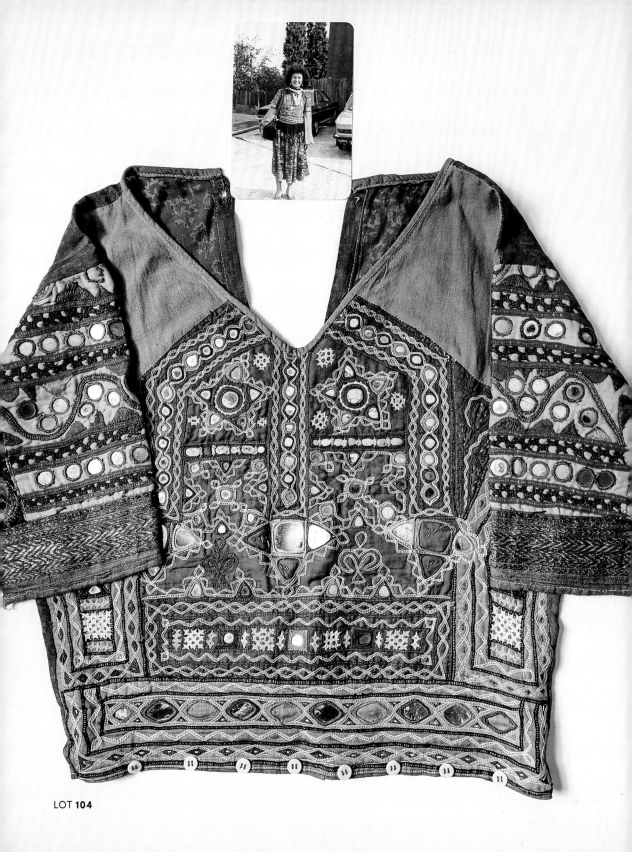

LOT **104**

# aroma of the beedi

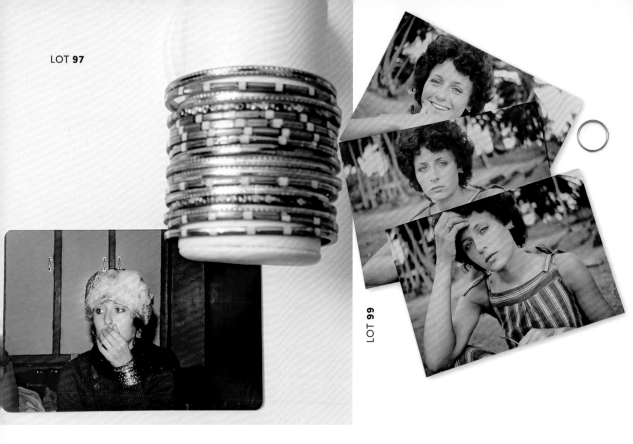

LOT **97**
## A SET OF INDIAN PLASTIC BANGLES AND PHOTOGRAPH
$5–$10 (WITHDRAWN)

On 27 November 1980, aged 25, I set off with an antiques-dealer boyfriend on my first, life-changing journey to India.

My journal entry for that day reads:

*"Arrive Bombay at 6am local time and make a good luck wish. Out of the plane we all troop onto an old bus which takes us ten yards to the waiting for customs etc and I think it's really hilarious. Have to wait two and a half hours to get through, lots of silly forms, and Indians running backwards and forwards and then someone knocks over the Custom man's desk by mistake and everything goes flying. All the Germans are getting stroppy – even the Indians who have just arrived say it's ridiculous, but I laugh and it's OK."*

These bangles were bought on that first trip. I never felt the urge to buy another set of plastic bangles – these pink and gold, and multicoloured bangles covered my every need, satisfied me completely and became a symbol of the massive shift in my view of the world and the core of my heart.

## LOT **98**

### *THE NEW STANDARD,* 9 DECEMBER 1980

$5–$10

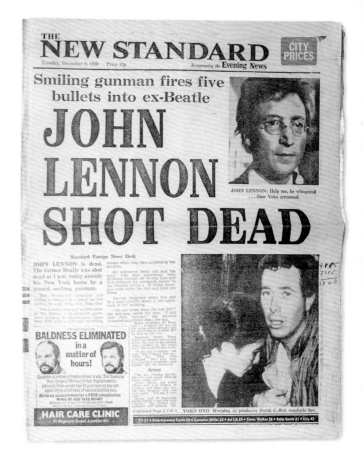

I remember 8 December 1980 very clearly, not because I was dreadfully sick with food poisoning, resting on a rope bed in a tiny hut on the foreshore of Kovalam beach in Kerala, southern India, but because it was the day I heard the news that John Lennon had been shot. Dead.

My diary entry reads: *"Knocked sideways by the news that John Lennon has been murdered outside his apartment in Manhattan. This is the biggest loss in musical history that I can ever imagine."*

A friend gave this newspaper to me on my return to London.

## LOT **99**

### 18CT GOLD WEDDING RING, c1900, WITH THREE PHOTOGRAPHS, JANUARY 1981

$100–$140

These photographs were taken in Tangalle, Sri Lanka, on my first trip to India and Sri Lanka. Although we weren't married, I was travelling with Geoff, an antiques-dealer boyfriend, and wore this wedding band. I felt it would offer me some protection from the harassment that, as a young woman embarking on a big adventure, I believed would occur. As it turned out, although this first trip was challenging in many ways, I generally felt safe, secure and accepted. This was the start of my love affair with India, and this ring now symbolises a form of unity I felt deep within me.

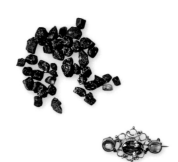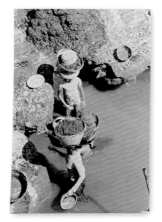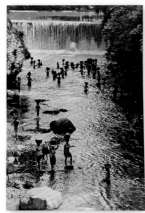

LOT **100**

**18CT GOLD BROOCH SET WITH A CEYLON SAPPHIRE AND TWO MOONSTONES, EARLY 1900s, PARCEL OF ROUGH (UNCUT) SAPPHIRES, AND TWO PHOTOGRAPHS, 1980**

$250–$300

The handmade brooch was probably made in what was known in those days as Ceylon. The loose sapphires probably originate from Inverell in Australia. I took these photographs in 1980 in the Rathnapura district of Sri Lanka.

I was becoming increasingly interested in gemstones, their origins, the processes of recovery and subsequent treatments. I decided to travel to Sri Lanka to see for myself the geography and method of recovery of the world-famous cornflower-blue sapphires. I learnt that, in Sri Lanka, there were two types of mining, underground mines – which, as a woman, I was not allowed to visit – and alluvial 'mining', where the gemstones are gathered in baskets from gem gravels in rivers. The gravels are handwashed to recover the gems.

It is amazing to think that the beautiful blue stone in the middle of this little brooch has been through all these, and many more, processes.

LOT **101**

**VINTAGE RAJASTHANI SKIRT AND AN INLAID ALABASTER BOX, AGRA, 1981, AND TWO PHOTOGRAPHS**

$20–$30

The inlaid box was the least expensive, yet still appealing and useful small item I could find to represent my first visit to the Taj Mahal. The embroidered green cotton skirt remains a constant when I'm packing for a trip to India (see Lot 190).

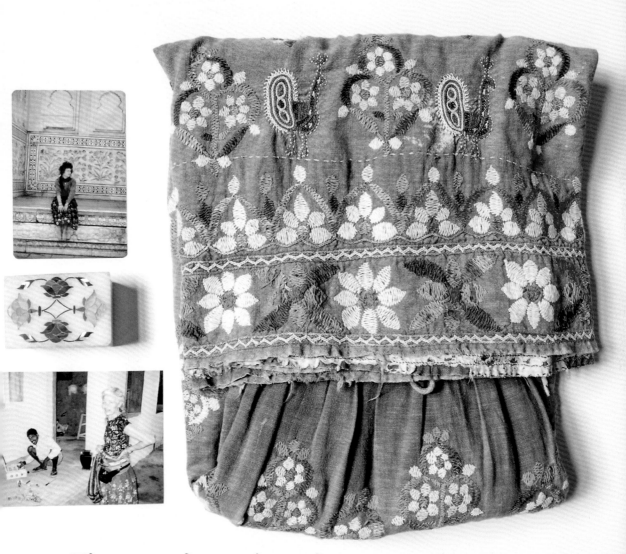

The embroidered green skirt remains a constant when I'm packing for India.

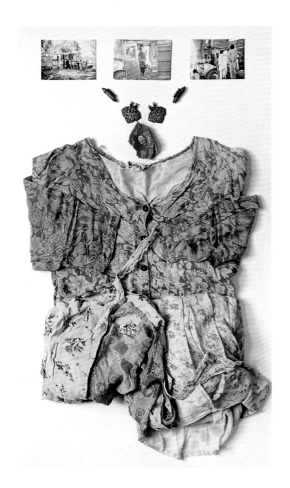

## LOT 102

### VARIOUS ITEMS OF INDIAN JEWELLERY, A VINTAGE DRESS, AND THREE PHOTOGRAPHS

$30–$50

This was the dress I was wearing whilst journeying on a local bus from Agra to Jaipur on a fateful day during my first time in India. Our trip was interrupted for several hours by a ghastly accident in which a truck, swerving in an attempt to miss an oncoming bus, had smashed into a tree. All road traffic was halted and we sat beside the road for hours as local people pulled out the driver, ambulances arrived and the bus was pushed back onto the road.

The only other tourists on the bus were a couple of Australian boys, public servants from Adelaide, who were on an extended trip during their one-year long-service leave. We chatted briefly and later, bumped into them whilst we were doing the rounds of Jaipur, before going our separate ways. I have no idea whether the driver survived.

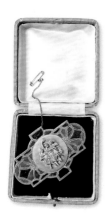

## LOT 103

### VICTORIAN SILVER BROOCH WITH CENTRAL CARTOUCHE DEPICTING THE THREE GRACES, c1900

$380–$450

Although this brooch was made in Scotland using locally quarried bloodstone and carnelian, I bought it in an antiques shop in Bombay on my first visit to India in 1980. It may seem odd that I kept an antique Scottish brooch as a souvenir from India, yet now I am married to a Scotsman and our 1997 marriage ceremony was held in Jaipur.

Life works in mysterious ways, and I don't believe in coincidences.

## LOT **104**

### COTTON GUJARATI KUTCH EMBROIDERED BLOUSE, 1981, AND PHOTOGRAPH, 1982 (SHOWN ON PAGE 124)

$50–$70

The photograph, taken in London, shows me in a Biba T-shirt under a blouse made up from old scraps of embroidery that I had found the previous year on an old wooden cart in the main street of Jaipur. It features mirror work, called abhla, and different stitching techniques, including chain stitch and blanket stitch. The machine stitching was done by an old man, who, on the side of the road, with his trusty treadle Singer sewing machine, converted the scraps into a wearable garment for me.

## LOT **105**

### PLAYER'S NAVY CUT CIGARETTE TIN, c1900, WITH SIX BOXES OF CHEETA MATCHES, 1981

$20–$40

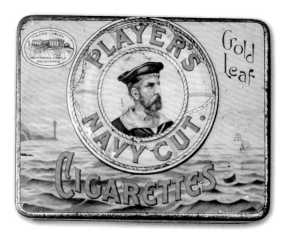

The sense of smell is surely one of the most evocative. I am always entranced by the aroma of the beedi, the traditional Indian cigarette made with tobacco rolled into a leaf and bound with a tie of, often, deep-pink cotton thread. Returning to London from my first trip to India, my duty-free cigarette allowance was made up of two large bundles containing 400 beedis. These Cheeta matches were a gift from the excited beedi-wallah, whose main trade was selling individual beedi sticks to the dusty street dwellers. The poorest folk are often the most generous.

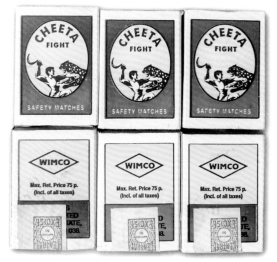

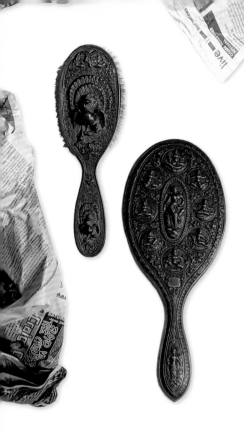

## LOT 106
### INDIAN SILVER HAIRBRUSH AND MIRROR, c1880
$350–$450

Vestiges of another world, other times and other lives. If only these pieces could talk, what stories they could tell. Their design shows the merging of Anglo and Indian influence. They would have been made in India during the days of the Raj, when wealthy women's long tresses would be groomed with hairbrushes made with horse-hair bristles.

In January 1980, the price of silver hit an all-time high of about US$50 an ounce. This was as much as 10 times what it had been for some 30 years, and it sparked a feeding frenzy in the markets, the like of which I had never seen before and hope never to see again. London's silver dealers, dressed in their long black overcoats and hats, would be seen bustling around the markets, scales in one hand and big swag bags in the other.

We lowly antiques dealers, those of us with an aesthetic eye and a love of what the pieces represented, were appalled, outraged and disgusted at what we were witnessing.

In Hatton Garden, the lines outside bullion centres represented an annihilation of history, a mass destruction of treasures. People queued up along the pavements, smashing up Georgian tea services, beautifully embossed trays and exquisitely enamelled dressing-table sets, whose value as scrap far surpassed their value as an item. To me, it was obscene and mortifying – and the first time I became aware of the commodification of raw materials over art and culture.

I rescued these two treasures during that time. They were due to be smashed – the mirror, brush and shellac would be discarded, and the peacock and supernatural female apsaras would be crushed and melted into ingots. I could not let this happen. These beauties subsequently were wrapped in newspaper dated 11 June 2006, in preparation for a house move. The move turned into a major restoration, which meant that three boxes were only recently unpacked, including the one containing this hairbrush and mirror.

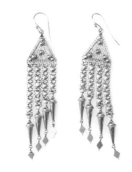

## LOT **107**
## PAIR OF HANDMADE 22CT GOLD EARRINGS,
## c2000, AND PHOTOGRAPH, 1981
$1500–$1800

The photograph was taken after my first trip to India and
just prior to my second. I am wearing a blue woollen jumper
handknitted by my grandmother, which I subsequently
gave to a Nepalese boy who acted as a porter and became
a friend on a trek I took in the Annapurna Range of the
Himalayas later that year. In the photograph, I'm wearing
what were my favourite fringed silver-gilt and turquoise
earrings, which I later sold. My choice in earrings has
remained the same; these were made in Rajasthan and
purchased in Mumbai sometime in the early 2000s.

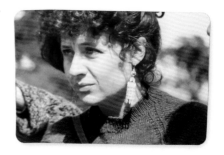

## LOT **108**
## SILVER AND ENAMEL CIGARETTE CASE,
## AND ENAMEL POWDER COMPACT, c1920
$800–$1200

Back in England, the street markets became my world. I was living
with a gay friend, Nick, in leafy Wembley, and working amongst the
misfits of society – people of all ethnicities, ages, backgrounds, sexual
orientations, economic levels and political persuasions. We were
a melting pot of loyal, crazy, desperate, hardworking, fun-loving
people. It was in this environment that I was discovering my eye,
honing my craft by absorbing information from all those around me.

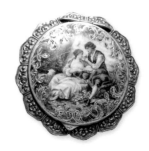

Many of my close friends, people with whom I socialised
and worked, were the gay boys. They were such fun, so
welcoming, accepting, kind and generous. These boys had an
eye for enamelware, and I would search for quality examples
of enamelled art deco calling-card cases, Vesta matchboxes
and cigarette cases for them. This example of an enamel case
imitating a snakeskin was, however, never offered for sale,
as it fitted well into my love of items inspired by the natural
world. It still evokes memories of my boys, though.

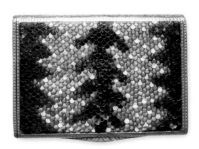

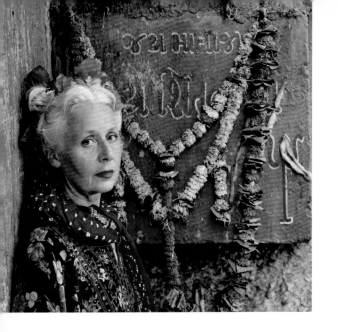

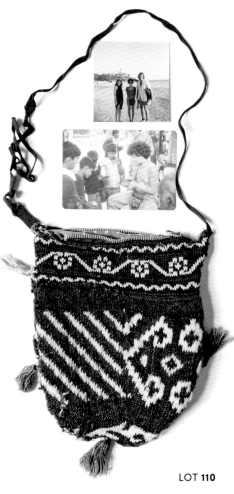

**LOT 109**

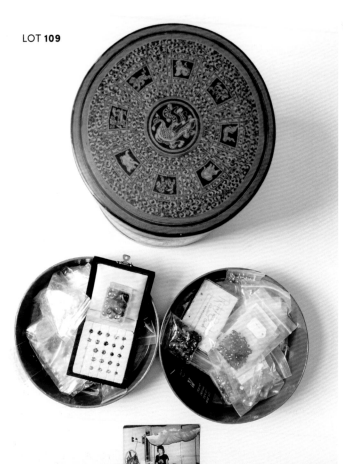

**LOT 110**

## LOT 109

### THREE-TIERED BURMESE LACQUER BOX CONTAINING LOOSE GEMSTONES, AND PHOTOGRAPH, 1981

$3000–$3500

Why is it that whenever dealers buy a piece of jewellery with a stone missing, their box of spares never has one to fit the setting? This is my gemstones box, filled to the brim with all manner of gorgeous, multicoloured, multifaceted loose gemstones. Amongst them is the vintage rectangular cardboard box, optimistically labelled 'RUBIES' in bold blue letters. I picked this up for a song many years later at a deceased-estate auction in Adelaide. The 'rubies' turned out to be rough garnet crystals, all uncut. Although of little value, they are somehow more appealing to me as I wonder who their previous owner was and whether they thought they had serious treasure in that little box. Such a great reminder that you can't take it with you. Life is the treasure – although a little bit of optimism goes a very long way.

Whilst I was in Burma (Myanmar) for a week in 1981 – the statutory time quota for tourists at that time of military rule – I traded the three-tier lacquer box for a small portable radio. I learnt from a ruby merchant in Mandalay (a wonderful woman who took me under her wing) that the closer you get to the source of gemstones, the more fakes you are offered on the street.

The photograph shows the standard of tourist accommodation back then. Quite literally, there were rats running over the bed.

## LOT 110

### WOVEN BAG (ORIGIN UNKNOWN), AND TWO PHOTOGRAPHS, 1980

$5–$10

This woven bag came to me from a jumble sale in the late 1970s. I have no idea of its age and origin, but was immediately attracted to its roughness and toughness, bold design and jaunty tassels. I lined it, added a zipper and strap, and it became my personal travelling bag on my first trip to India. In one photograph, taken in early December 1980, I'm wearing it on a Trivandrum beach in Kerala. In the other, I'm in Jaipur in conversation with a group of shoe-shine boys. On that first trip to India, before I came to understand the multi levels of (self) employment, I felt guilty having someone else clean my shoes, so I was trying to negotiate paying for a small amount of polish so I could do it myself. The boys were very confused and clearly I was, too.

## LOT 111
## VINTAGE BLACK LEATHER BELT, AND PRESS CLIPPING, 1981
$1–$5 (WITHDRAWN)

The first time I was ever stopped on the street to be photographed was here, in the spring of 1981. I was strolling along the Kings Road in Chelsea, chomping on an apple and dressed in a 1960s stripy number, teamed with my favourite white cowboy boots and black leather belt. Nobody seemed to worry that I had chipmunk cheeks full of apple as a photograph was hastily taken.

Jean Dobson, the author of the piece, wrote: *"Forget about the so-called dictates of fashion, these girls are each stamping their own personality and flair on how they wear the mini."*

This belt has been a staple part of my wardrobe for decades.

In 1998, I was with my husband and nine-year-old twin girls on a flight from India to London and, as we were passing through security checks at Heathrow, each member of the group was allocated bags to carry. Tash was given the black wheelie, which contained various items, including the belt. On reaching our destination, we realised the wheelie was missing. I reported the lost bag, listing all the items it contained, and put it out of my mind. Accidents happen, although I must admit I was really pissed off at losing my treasured black belt, the least valuable, yet most significant item in the bag.

Some six months later, completely out of the blue, a van drove up to my place in London and delivered the wheelie bag. Most of the things that had been inside were missing, but the black belt, of little value, remained! Happy days.

Tash subsequently borrowed the belt for many of her teenage years. We call it a long-term loan. It was returned to me in two parts. This is of no consequence, as it only adds to the significance of the item, which serves as a physical connection between me and my daughter.

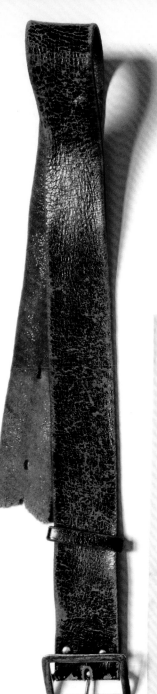

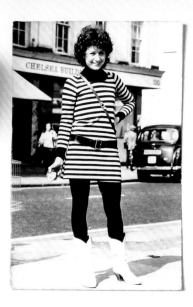

AS THE TEMPERATURE RISES...SO DOES THE HEMLINE

Photo Shows: Striped dress belted on the hipbones.

50                                    810409/01

See Companion Pictures

Associated Newspapers
Copyright

# *Femail* FOCUS ON YESTERDAY'S EYE-CATCHING LEG SHOW

## As the temperature rises
## ...so does the hemline

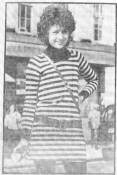

Striped dress belted on the hipbone.

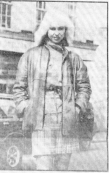

Highland kilt and zipper leather jacket.

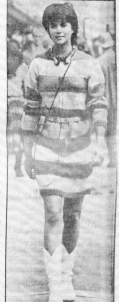

Home-knitted sweater dress with hi-fi accessories.

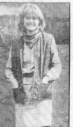

The Wild West way, with an arresting kerchief.

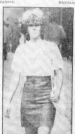

Hip-hugging skirt and short-sleeved top and short hair.

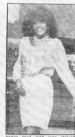

Pencil skirt with long-sleeved blouse.

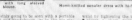

THE temperature rose all over Britain yesterday and — as these pictures show — not just because of the sunny weather.

For, after years of argument — will it, won't it, the Mini is positively back. Had forgot about the old version that made your mother swing in the Sixties.

On the hottest day of the year with London and the South-East having the highest temperatures of 80 F, the Mail sent its photographers on to the streets all over Britain to catch how to-day's girls are shedding their coats and jeans for the sensational leg show. And, to the delight of most men, they're doing it with a panache and speed that's pure fashion. Forget about the so-called dictates of fashion — these girls are each stamping their own personality and flair on how they wear the Mini.

This time the hemlines are thigh level and coloured tights are teamed with cowboy boots. Or flat-heeled shoes balance the tough-line. But, as in any new craze — and the Mini will be just that if we have a hot summer — how its worn will change. It is certainly going to be seen with a portable hi-fi and headphones — as in the big picture right.

But if you are turning up your skirt, or belting up a sweater dress shorter than last week or knitting a jumper with a thigh band, take time off to study your legline and in particular your thighs. The Mini is essentially a young style that doesn't suit everybody.

Here's how you can get the instant Mini look:

● belt a long sweater at the hipbone
● make a pleated skirt higher at the waist by tightening the buckle fastening
● blouse a frock dress at the waist baggily over the belt, wear it with a Western waistcoat, neck scarf and fringed boots.

If the last time around the Mini was flamboyant, aggressive and mini-skirt wearers aoded it to pay the difference this time is the relaxed way it is being worn, typifying the new cool approach.

Which is more than can be said of the delighted males passing.

JEAN DOBSON

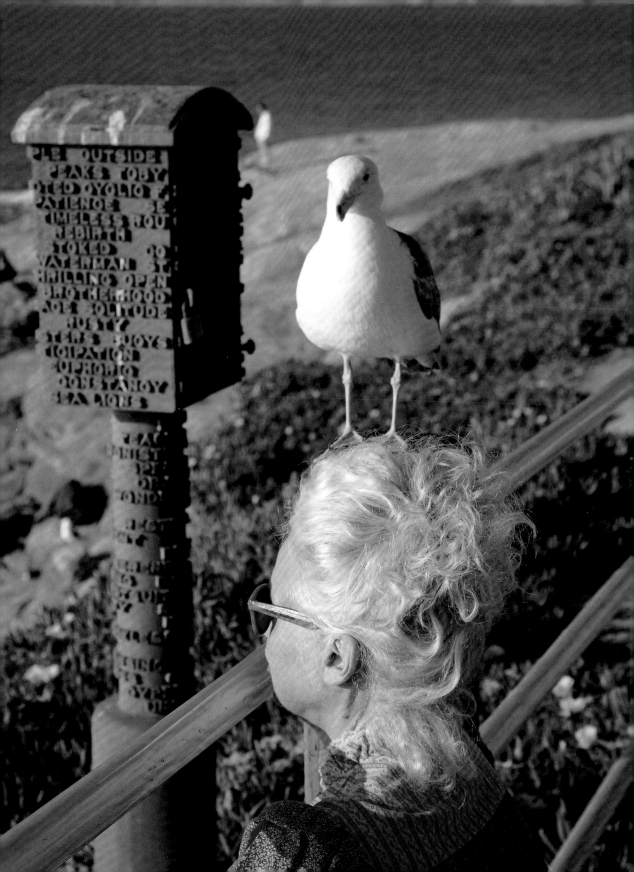

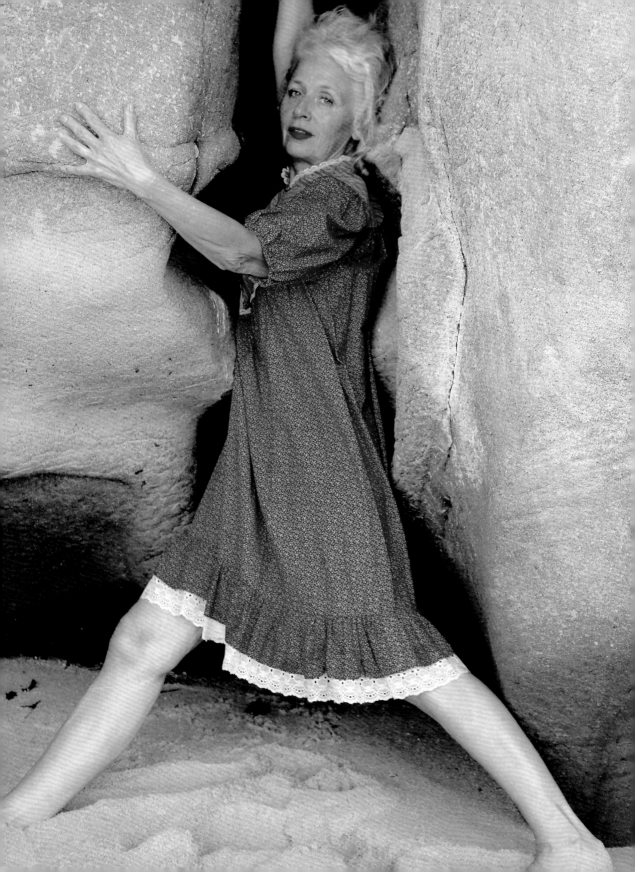

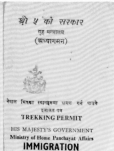

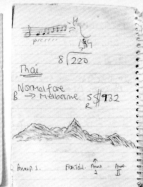

### Trekking Permit document (centre top)

श्री ५ को सरकार
गृह मन्त्रालय
(अध्यागमन)

The bearer has been granted permission by His Majesty's Government to trek to and from the places mentioned overleaf via main routes. He/she must, however, keep twentyfive miles of the northern borders of Nepal.

The Ministry of Home Panchayat Affairs appreciate any such courtesy and assistance as he/she may stand in need of by the Anchaladhish (Zonal Commissioner), Sahayak Anchaladhish (Assistant Zonal Commissioner), Pramukh Zila Adhikari (Chief District Officer), Check-Post and local people concerned at his/her own expense in the course of trekking.

नेपाल भिक्षा स्वास्थ्यभर भ्रमण गर्न पाउने
इजाजत पत्र
TREKKING PERMIT
HIS MAJESTY'S GOVERNMENT
Ministry of Home Panchayat Affairs
IMMIGRATION
KATHMANDU

7

### Notebook (top right)

KATHMANDU → POKHRA.
12ᵗʰ Thursday Nov 1981.

Thai
Normal fare
B → Melbourne  S$932
R

Annap. S.  Fishtail  Annap I  Annap II

---

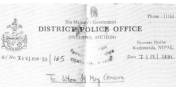

His Majesty's Government
### DISTRICT POLICE OFFICE
(INTERPOL SECTION)

Phone : 11162

Hanuman Dhoka
Kathmandu, NEPAL.

Ref. No: I 12/038-39/165        Date: 1.13.1981.

To Whom It May Concern

This is to Certify that British national Miss Sarah Jane Adams bearer of passport no- L 142 982 A has reported to this office about the loss of down sleeping bag and down jacket on 30th Nov. 1981 in the bus route of Pokhara at Kathmandu.

Further police Investigation is on process.

A.S.I.
Police Officer
[Tika Ram Shipwal]

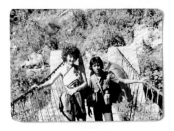

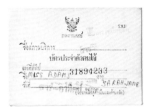

MISS ADAM   31894233
SARAHJANE

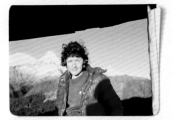

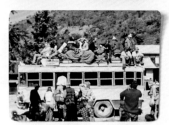

---

### Letter (bottom left)

VALLEY VIEW HOTEL
KATHMANDU
NEPAL.

POLICY NO 600348

1st Dec 1981

Dear Sir,

I am writing to report that I had a sleeping bag costing £65.00, and a down jacket, costing £60.00, stolen from my rucksack on 29th Nov 1981. My insurance policy was taken from 27th Oct 1981 for 6 months. I will be travelling throughout Asia for this period, so hope that any further communication with you can be made with my mother.

MRS D. M. ADAMS
YORK HOUSE
ST LEONARDS
TICKHILL
DONCASTER, DN11 9HX
YORKS ENGLAND.

Tel. 0302 742089.

Because the police system here in Nepal is very unreliable, I have here photocopies of my insurance claim form and the document from the police, and will send you these, rather than the originals. Would it be possible for you to confirm to my mother that these have arrived within the statutory 28 days?

### Letter (bottom centre)

I am unable to enclose receipts for the articles stolen because I don't have them with me here in Nepal. It is possible that my mother has kept them, although I can not be certain of this.

The details of the loss of the items is as follows:-

I was travelling on a local bus from Pokhara to Kathmandu on 29th Nov 1981. Originally I was sitting on the top of the bus with my rucksack, but when the bus went through a police check, everyone on the top of the bus was made to sit inside. The bus was very crowded & the conductor said that all the luggage had to remain in the roof to make room for more passengers. Because I was in the countryside, miles from anywhere & with no possibility of catching another bus, I had to oblige. Every time the bus stopped, I got out to check that the rucksack was still on top. The journey lasted about 9 hours, during which the bus picked up many local Nepalese people, some of which were by this time sitting on the top of the bus again.

When I got back to my hotel in Kathmandu I see above at the top of bus later I noticed no rucksack in anticipa-

### Letter (bottom right)

that the entire contents had been taken out and replaced untidily, and that my back down sleeping bag and back down jacket had been stolen. Obviously someone had gone through the rucksack in between stops, and had got off the bus before it reached Kathmandu.

The following day I enquired at the bus station in Kathmandu as to whether the 2 items had been handed in, not surprisingly the answer was no.

Then I went and reported the theft to the police station. Police officer Tika Ram Shizwal came back & searched my hotel room and saw that the sleeping bag + jacket were not there. However, the detachable hood of the jacket was not taken because it was packed in a side pocket of the rucksack and was obviously not noticed.

I will be able to contact you via my mother, if you need any further information could you please get in touch with her.

My London address on the insurance policy is 17, HAZLEDENE RD, CHISWICK, W4 3JB, LONDON.

Yours sincerely,
Sarah Jane Adams

---

# CHAPTER 8

# I made the move

**FIVE PACKS OF PLAYING CARDS (ALL COMPLETE): EDWARDIAN DOUBLE DECK FEATURING ORIENTAL CARPET DESIGN, c1910; RATHDOWN CLUB DECK DEPICTING INDIAN ATOP AN ELEPHANT, c1920; JUNK CARD GAME, LIMITED EDITION, 1980–81; WILLIE RUSHTON'S PACK OF ROYALS, WITH CARICATURES OF THE BRITISH ROYAL FAMILY, 1995; THE NATURAL WORLD PLAYING CARD COLLECTION: GEMSTONES OF THE WORLD, 1999**

$100–$150

How much of life is luck and how much is destiny?

I was back in Portobello "selling your wares on the street corner", as my father so delightfully put it. I was used to seeing faces I recognised, so when two scruffy young men wandered past, I greeted them, trying my best to remember where I had seen them before. Turns out they were the two Aussies I had met the previous year, when we were all on the fateful bus travelling from Agra to Jaipur. The boys had spent several months cycling through Europe and now had a few weeks in London before returning, via India, to Australia. They stayed with me and a girlfriend, with whom my imminent trip to India was planned.

The boys, on hearing that we were making a trip to Asia, extended an invitation to us, suggesting we continue on to Australia. They kindly lent us equipment for our forthcoming trek in Nepal, including feather-down jackets, boots and medicine.

I knew nothing more of Australia than what I'd learnt in 'O' level Geography. What I did know was that I was intrigued by one of these boys, and very keen to see him again. Returning the borrowed trekking gear in person seemed a perfect reason to continue on to Australia, so we accepted their invitation.

Whether or not it was written in the cards, the future held two marriages between the four of us.

*The future held two marriages between the four of us.*

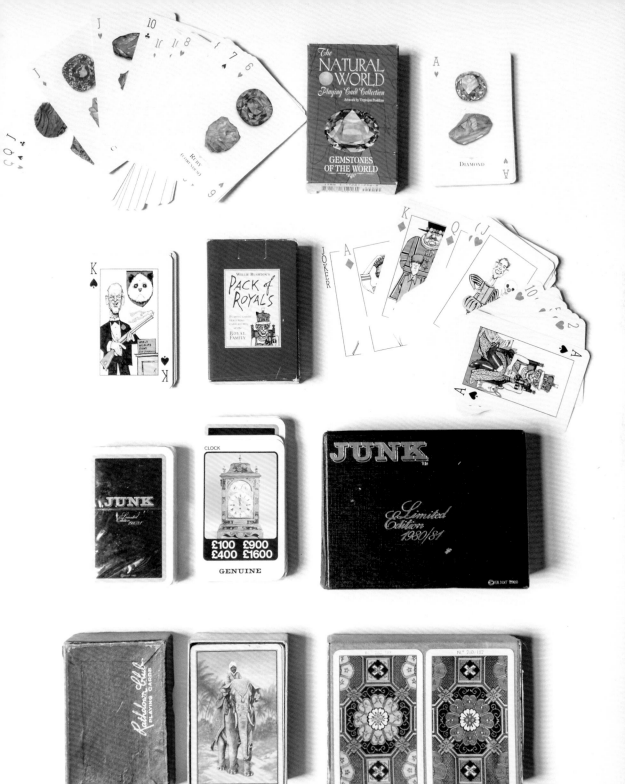

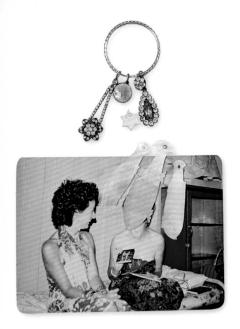

## LOT 113
## 9CT GOLD HOOP EARRING WITH ASSORTED CHARMS, AND PHOTOGRAPH, 1981
$50–$100

In October 1981, I arrived with my girlfriend on my second trip to India. We spent a few days in Delhi with the Australian boys, who were en route back to Adelaide.

The photograph was taken in Paharganj, Delhi, shortly before we left for Nepal. St Christopher is known to Catholics as the patron saint of travellers. The bangles I'm wearing are also seen in Lots 95 and 97. In this image, my earring also features a Victorian horn of plenty coral charm, subsequently sold. The individual charms shown here include three 19th-century Chinese mother-of-pearl carved gaming counters and two Georgian paste and silver earrings.

## LOT 114
## A BOX OF 10 MINIATURE ORIENTAL PERFUMES, 1981
$10–$20

This little box of 'oriental perfumes' was selected by me in late 1981, in a very small shop in the Paharganj market area in Delhi. Although the shop was no bigger than a garden shed, the experience of the ritual, passion and knowledge the vendor clearly had for these exotic oils stays with me to this day. The importance of loving what you do, having a knowledge and an empathy for the product you are offering – these are characteristics I applied to my life and specifically as an antique-jewellery dealer. For me, the most tantalising fragrances in this little box are not the traditional Musk, Zinnia and Orchid, but the Oil of Soil and Amber.

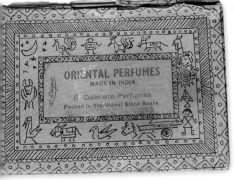

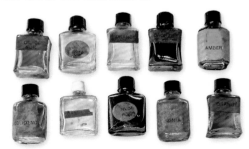

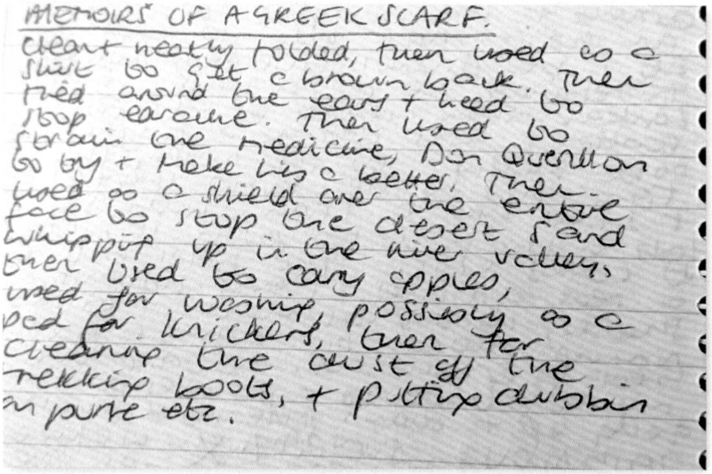

MEMOIRS OF A GREEK SCARF.

Clean, neatly folded, then used as a sheet to get a broken back. Then tied around the ears + head to keep earache. Then used to strain the medicine, Don Quentin to try + make his a better. Then used as a shield over the entire face to stop the desert sand whipped up in the River valley, then used to carry apples, used for washing, possibly as a pad for knickers, then for cleaning the dust off the trekking boots, + putting dubbin on boots etc.

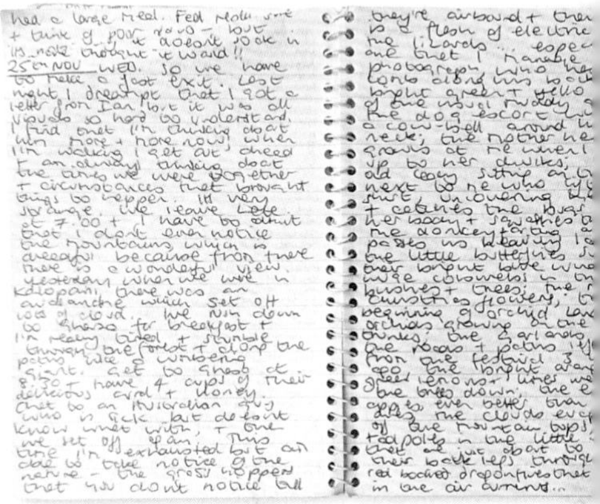

## LOT 115

# DIARY OF TRAVELS IN NEPAL AND OTHER EPHEMERA, 1981

NCV (WITHDRAWN)

The photograph on page 140 shows the diary opened on 12 November (followed by 25 and 29 November 1981 shown here).

My girlfriend and I spent three weeks in Nepal, during which time we made the trek from Pokhara to Jomsom amidst the spectacular Annapurna Ranges. At the end of the trek, we took a local bus from Pokhara back to Kathmandu, commencing our journey atop the roof with all the luggage, only moving inside later as spaces became available. On arrival in Kathmandu I realised that pretty much everything had been stolen from my rucksack, including all the Aussie boys' trekking equipment.

In order to claim travel insurance, I had to report the incident to the local police. The police officer repeatedly asked me what else had I lost. An expensive camera? A radio? Jewellery? Anything else of high value? Over the course of four days, I repeatedly told him no, no, no. Eventually, exasperated, he issued me with my letter. Only when I arrived in Australia did I realise that the officer had wanted me to make a higher (fraudulent) claim so he could receive a hefty 'baksheesh' payment (bribe) for his services.

Such a naive traveller, with still so much to learn. These days, I only take out health insurance when travelling.

One extract, written in Nepal, is 'Memoirs of a Greek scarf'. Here, I describe nine of the various uses of an item I had bought in Greece in 1975, seen being worn as a 'shirt' in Lot 85, and as a neck scarf in Lot 104.

I like to think that The Greek Scarf continued to have many further uses in its next life, thanks to the person who removed it from my rucksack.

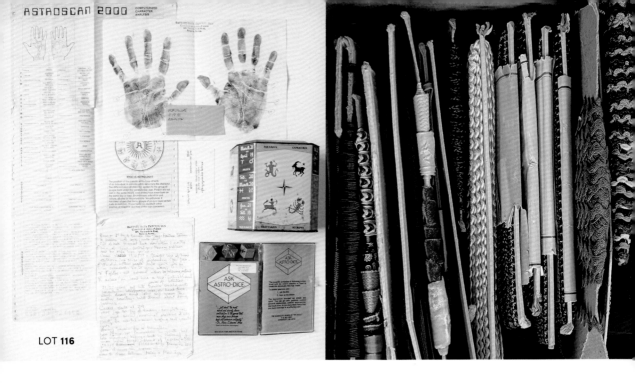

LOT 116

## LOT 116

### TIN WITH ZODIAC DECORATION, A GAME OF ASTRO-DICE, AND OTHER PARAPHERNALIA

$50–$70

The first time I had my palm read was in Rangoon, Burma, in 1981. My girlfriend summarised what was said. A marriage was predicted – one that wouldn't last.

## LOT 117

### A BOX OF ASSORTED VINTAGE CORDS AND BRAIDS, DATING FROM THE EARLY 1900s

$60–$80

We arrived in Adelaide, where life was slower, calmer and generally more laid back than the frenetic pace of London in the 1980s. Once settled, I had plenty of time to revisit my passion for sewing, redesigning and restitching garments. I also attended auctions looking for antique jewels, clothes and any items I could on-sell to support myself whilst in Australia. I quickly fell in with the dealers, attending all the auctions and antiques fairs.

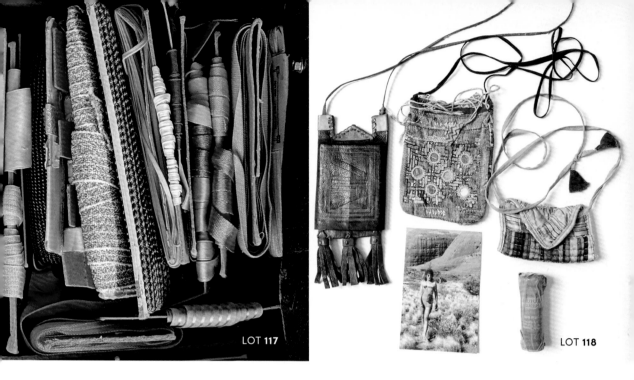

LOT 117

LOT 118

There were 'trash and treasure' markets – one where I picked up a heavy and dependable old sewing machine. I bought these 'cords and braids of all descriptions' (as they were catalogued) at a deceased-estate auction. For 40 years, this box has provided me with all the scraps I have needed for decorating clothes, gifts and presentations for all occasions for my two children.

LOT 118

## THREE SMALL BAGS AND A PHOTOGRAPH

$5–$10

I like to travel light. Before the days of mobile phones, unless I was carrying jewellery, my daily essentials fitted into a very small bag, which I always wore slung across the body. The small bag on the right, also shown being worn in the photograph in Lot 125, has been with me since my early 20s and now contains a canister of holy Ganges water collected in Varanasi in 2003.

The photograph, taken at Uluru in Australia, shows me using the mirrored Indian purse and wearing an Indian orange sarong. On these early trips, I explored much of Australia, where, in cities and country towns, I also scoured antiques and antique-jewellery shops.

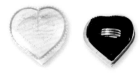

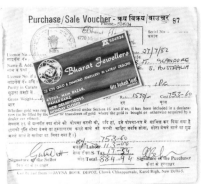

LOT **119**

## A 22CT GOLD WEDDING BAND WITH RED ENAMEL DETAIL IN INDIAN JEWELLERY BOX, 1982

$250–$300

For a number of reasons, one of the Aussie boys and I decided to marry. Given our serendipitous meeting and the fact that we continued to travel to India, it seemed only natural that the ring be made in the country I had come to love. The ring seen here is in its original box, along with a receipt dated 27 July 1982 from Bharat Jewellers, New Delhi. The ring was made to my exact specifications, with three gold stripes separated by two bands of red enamel.

Bharat Jewellers remains in the same location today as it was in 1982.

LOT **120**

## THEWA-WORK BOX MADE IN PRATABGARH, RAJASTHAN, 1800s, A PAIR OF EARRINGS, AND WEDDING-INVITATION CARDS

$500–$650

We bought the wedding invitations in Delhi. They feature a Pahari miniature of Radha and Krishna. The silver-gilt and green-enamel box, also depicting lovers, contains the pictured pair of earrings together with a 'Total Weight' ticket from the time of our wedding showing 59kg. My weight remains the same today.

## LOT 121

### MOROCCAN WOOLLEN ZEMMOUR BERBER CARPET, 1981, AND BALINESE JAKPAC JACKET

$30–$50

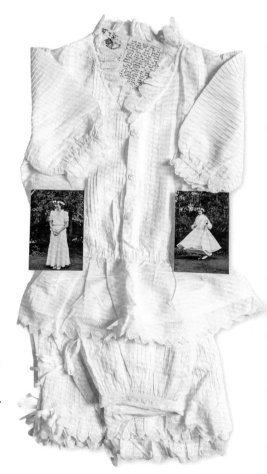

Prior to our wedding, we spent time in Morocco. I had travelled through Bali and picked up about 20 Jakpac jackets. Made with brightly coloured heavy cotton, they had arty patches with instructions on how to turn them into backpacks or bags. They were the epitome of cool, hadn't yet hit London and I was planning to sell most of them in the markets. Because we had nowhere in England to leave our stuff, they came with us in our rucksacks to Morocco. Travelling through the Atlas Mountains, I met a Berber family, weavers of traditional Moroccan carpets. We swapped all 20 jackets for two of their carpets. These graced my floors until they became threadbare, and now one remains as a winter covering for the floor in my sunroom. The jacket pictured here is a later purchase from the same era.

## LOT 122

### HANDMADE WHITE COTTON BLOUSE AND SKIRT, 1982

$20–$40

An imminent wedding in the English autumn with not a clue what to wear... On a stopover in Thailand in mid-1982, I was wandering through the street markets of Khao San in Bangkok, when I spotted this blouse. Handmade crisp cotton, featuring pin-tucks with broderie anglaise trimming, its price was right and I knew it would be absolutely perfect. I spoke with the stallholder and explained that I was soon to be married so I needed a full outfit. She took my waist measurement and within a few days I had a skirt, which, combined with the blouse, made the perfect dress. I took it back to Adelaide and asked my travelling-companion girlfriend, who was heading back to London, to take it with her. It was too tricky to keep such a thing a secret unless it was out of the way.

On my return to England, I found the Edwardian topcoat (seen being worn at the wedding reception in the photograph opposite), made from fine Kashmiri wool, in the Portobello Road. It was heavy, beautiful quality and a perfect combination with my Victorian-inspired dress. Knowing I would never wear it again after the wedding, I sold it in Sydney for a hefty profit, shortly after we returned to Australia as a married couple.

## PAIR OF ART DECO PLATINUM AND DIAMOND EARRINGS, IN BOX, c1920

$2500–$2800

In September 1982, in Fishbourne, Sussex, I married my Australian husband.

Some years before, in the early days of my antiques business, I had purchased these earrings from a dealer at an antiques fair. In those days, I would drive my Hillman Imp (bought for £50 from a generous friend) the length and breadth of the country, scouring the trade fairs held in local church halls, village community centres and the like.

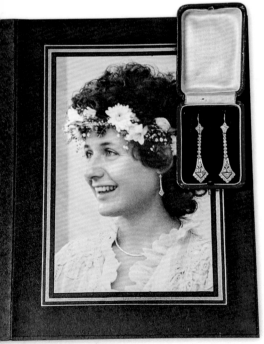

I remember spotting these beauties from a distance, glinting at me as they hung on an old lace tablecloth amongst an array of costume trinkets at the back of a stall. I asked the price. "Twelve pounds," said the lady. Without requesting the obligatory 'trade discount', I hurriedly paid the price and scampered off to give the earrings a closer inspection. Indeed, they were 'real' – genuine art deco diamond earrings.

My apprenticeship had been on the streets of London, ducking and diving, wheeling and dealing, learning from my elders – the old-timers who had been forging a living by using their wits, their 'eye', their knowledge and their banter. These special earrings represent a major breakthrough for me, not only as a bargain, but as confirmation that I was on my way to learning about gemstones and fine jewellery, and honing my aesthetic. I knew I had found my path. My life would be an adventure, rewarding in so many varied ways.

## 18CT GOLD ART NOUVEAU RING SET WITH SAPPHIRES, DESIGNED BY ARCHIBALD KNOX FOR LIBERTY, c1895

$3000–$3300 (WITHDRAWN)

I had found this ring in Bermondsey market in 1980 – a rare and special piece of jewellery. My best friend in the world coveted it, jokingly requesting I leave it to him in my will.

HIV/AIDS (a condition that at the time no one really understood but which was constantly discussed) was terrifying the gay community. That friend was one of the first to be taken by this dreadful virus. The photograph here shows me at my wedding reception with my dearest friends, many subsequently tragically lost as their immune systems were gradually destroyed, with little treatment available and devastating consequences.

My wedding to an Australian was bittersweet. I was leaving London to settle in a country a huge distance from Portobello Road, my umbilical cord to England, the place where all my friends were.

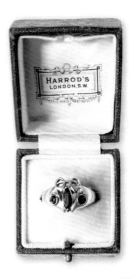

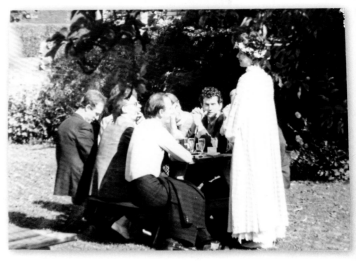

*My wedding to an Australian was bittersweet.*

## SUITCASE, COW BELL AND PHOTOGRAPH ALBUM

$20–$30

In my previous life, this battered blue suitcase had been my 'on the road' bag, as indicated by the stickers. The cow bell belonged to Pip Pyle, drummer of Hatfield and the North, and National Health, the two bands I'd been involved with in the 1970s and early 80s. The photograph taken at that time shows me wearing a bag that is part of Lot 118.

In 1983, after marrying an Aussie, I made the move from London to Adelaide. I had packed up my seemingly meagre belongings (which were, in fact, many small items of some considerable value) and stored them in my parents' roof whilst I was travelling. For some time, I had been living out of a suitcase or rucksack, but there were a few boxes and my old school trunk that needed to be sent to Australia.

Part of the reason we married was that my husband and I could see

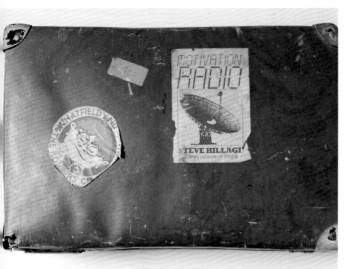
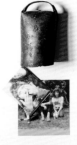
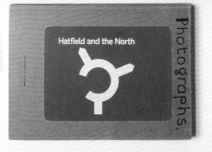

"good business opportunities". I had great contacts throughout the English antiques trade, and my new husband had a steady income from an Australian government job as a social worker.

The trend for antique stripped-pine furniture was at its height. In London I had already done some work in this area, stripping and restoring small pieces of furniture for personal use. One of my main jewellery suppliers, who lived in Yorkshire, was married to a furniture dealer whose sourcing reach covered the whole of the UK. It was a no-brainer that the four of us should work together and bring containers of furniture from the UK to Adelaide.

Our 'honeymoon' was spent travelling around the UK selecting stock. Everything went back to my supplier's rambling farmhouse in Yorkshire for storage and packing, along with my few boxes and school trunk.

The pink sticker on my blue suitcase is the inventory number for the import documentation on arrival into Australia. It reminds me of the thrilling, scary, incredible time when my few worldly possessions were packed into a couple of boxes, and then into a bigger, metal box, sailing on a massive container ship from my country of birth, to the other side of the world – and a new life.

LOT **126**

## A 22CT GOLD JAIPUR ENAMEL SPRINKLER FLASK, 1800s, AND SKETCH, 1983

$4500–$5000

The sketch I made of my new husband also shows details of the Adelaide auction houses, where on most days I could be found mooching around inspecting all the lots on offer. My apprenticeship in the markets of England and the streets of London served me well. I had amassed a broad and unique knowledge, and this, along with having a 'different' eye, enabled me to buy and sell all manner of items, frequently travelling interstate, and internationally, on buying and selling trips.

No one else attending the sale recognised this rosewater sprinkler, which was made during the time the Persian Mughal dynasty had control of what is now northern India.

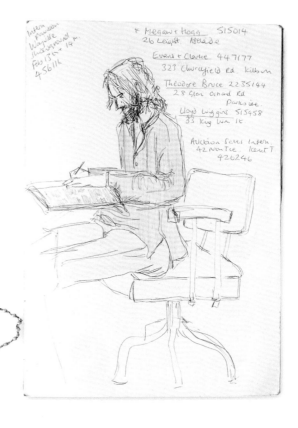

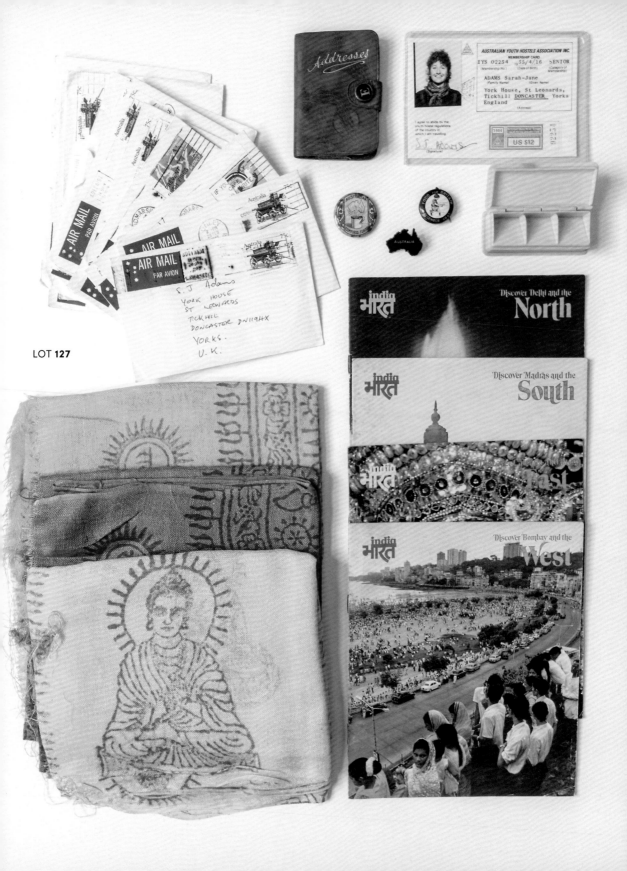

LOT **127**

## LOT 127

### SMALL LEATHER ADDRESS BOOK, THREE PINS, AND EPHEMERA INCLUDING LETTERS AND PHOTOGRAPHS, EARLY 1980s, AND CELLULOID STAMP CASE, c1900

$5–$10

To keep up the supply of antique jewellery to my newly found Australia-wide clients, I would need to make business trips to England three or four times a year. I signed up to an agency that organised courier flights. These were last-minute seats on international flights that were sold at a discounted price. The traveller was responsible for checking in an item of cargo, then hand-delivering it to a representative of the recipient company at the other end.

These flights came up at short notice, which suited me fine, as I had a great relationship with the antique-jewellery suppliers in London who held stock for me between trips. Couriers had to travel light, as the agency used our luggage allowance for the cargo. This was also OK, as I kept a few clothes with my friend in London. I really only needed a hand-luggage allowance. My bag came back to Australia full of antique jewellery, fully certified and ready for customs. Have bag, will travel.

The letters are from my Australian husband.

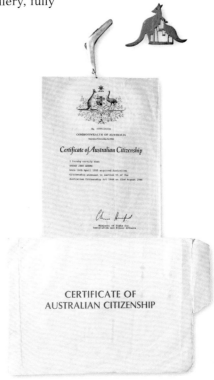

## LOT 128

### SILVER KANGAROO AND JOEY BROOCH, SILVER BOOMERANG-SHAPED PEN KNIFE AND GLOVE HOOK, AND COPY OF CERTIFICATE OF AUSTRALIAN CITIZENSHIP, 1986

$150–$250

By the time my Australian citizenship was approved, my international antique-jewellery business was well established. I had also already spent a great deal of time single-handedly redecorating my husband's house, where we lived together with a bunch of his friends.

I realised that, as the profits grew from my business, rather than allowing stock levels to rise exponentially (with the risk of them being either stolen or remaining unsold – thereby becoming 'dead stock'), bricks-and-

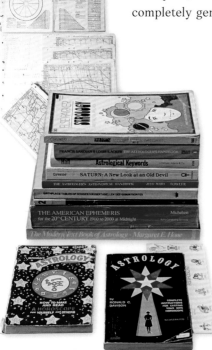

mortar was a more secure place to invest money. With the success of the business – combined with my husband's position as a public servant, allowing us to obtain a loan easily – we decided to purchase another property, a delightfully ramshackle worker's cottage in Bowden and Brompton, in those days, a 'desperate' suburb, which has now become completely gentrified.

## LOT 129
## COLLECTION OF BOOKS ON ASTROLOGY, 1970s–1980s
$30–$50

Life in Adelaide was the total opposite of the hustle and daily grind I had known in London. We planted veggies, had almonds and grapes growing plentifully in the backyard, and I had time to embark on the study of astrology. Unfortunately, the mathematical calculations they required meant that I only completed about 10 people's charts, but, for those of you who can read them, here are mine.

## LOT 130
## TIN BABY'S PERAMBULATOR TOY, c1940, AND FROZEN CHARLOTTE CHINA DOLL, c1900
$80–$120

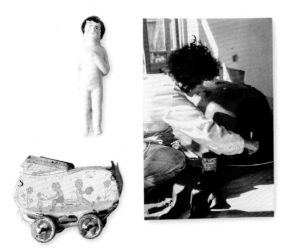

After a few years, I discovered I was pregnant. I wasn't sure how I felt about this turn of events, and don't even recall whether this pregnancy was planned or not. At the time I was heavily involved in major building projects, being the 'site manager' and general tradie on all the works being done on the cottage we had recently bought. I was demolishing walls, using all sorts of chemicals, lifting heavy lengths of timber and loads of bricks, and, perhaps not surprisingly, I suffered a miscarriage early in the pregnancy. I remember being sad but accepting. It was not the right time to have a child; I was due for a trip to England and realised that this was my opportunity to seriously consider my future.

## LOT 131

## VINTAGE PACK OF GLOWSTARS, WITH TWO HANDMADE BUTTON PINS AND ASSORTED EPHEMERA

$1–$5

There was this man from my past. He was an Aries like me – competitive, romantic, engaging, single-minded, challenging and exciting. We had an understanding. I collected egg cups; he, salt-and-pepper sets.

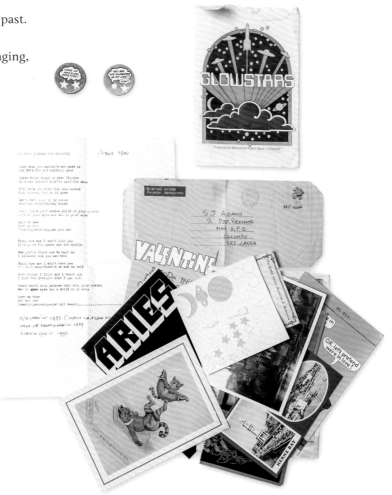

I reconnected with him in London, where, strolling with arms entwined along Kensington High Street, we were stopped by a woman who wanted to interview us. "Are you married?" she eagerly asked us. "Yes. But not to one another," was our simultaneous reply. It was eminently clear to me that on my return to Adelaide, my marriage would be over.

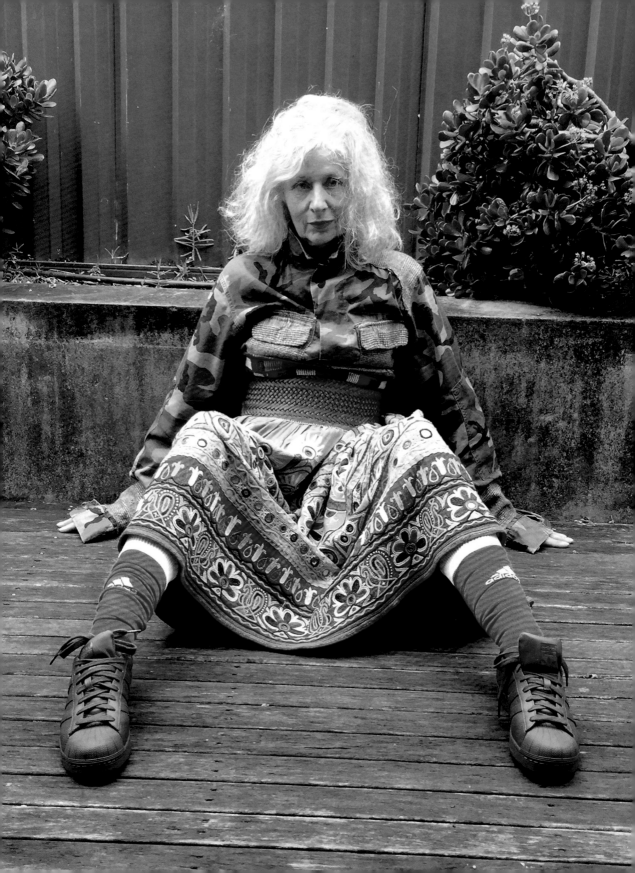

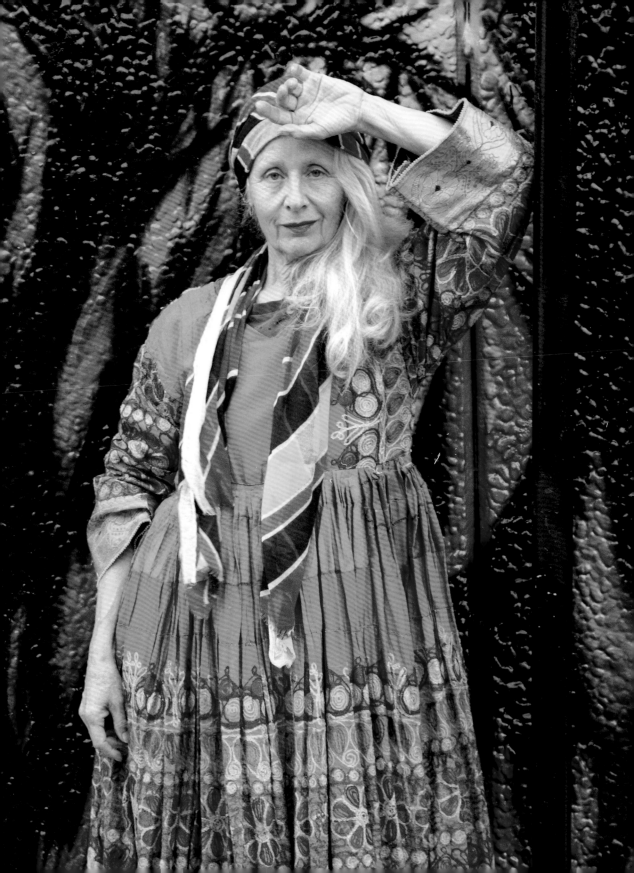

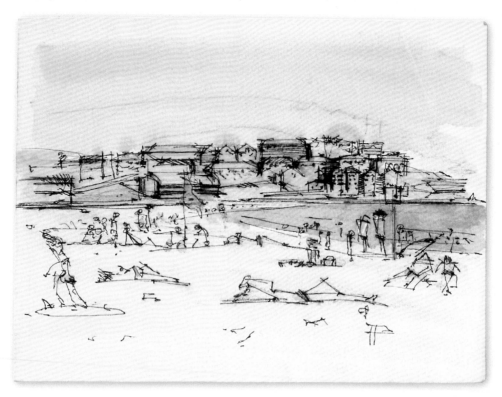

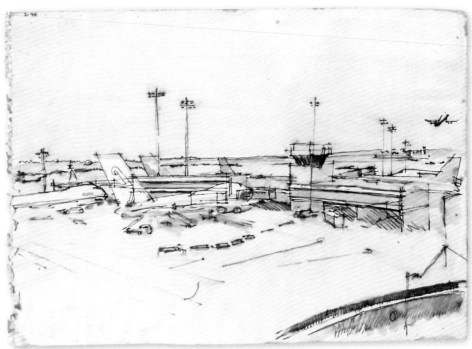

it feels
like
home

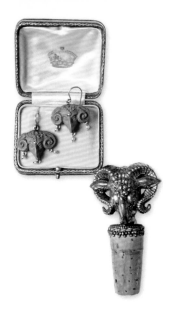

### LOT 132
### A PAIR OF HANDCARVED LAVA AND 15CT GOLD RAM'S-HEAD EARRINGS, IN BOX, c1860, AND ELECTRO-PLATED NICKEL SILVER (EPNS) RAM'S-HEAD BOTTLE STOPPER, c1920
$500–$600

By the end of 1987, this Aries (Ram) was divorced, had left pretty much everything in Adelaide behind and had moved to Sydney, where I was in the process of rediscovering who I was. Alone again, naturally.

### LOT 133
### 'SARAH JANE' HMSS NAME BROOCH IN BOX, CHESTER, 1900
$40–$60

Name brooches were produced in England for about 40 years, from the late 1800s to the early 1900s. The pieces were generally made in silver, occasionally with gold detail. They were mainly popular amongst the working classes, where they were given as sentimental gifts. As manufacturing techniques improved, jewellery, trinkets and keepsakes were becoming increasingly available and more affordable. Often these were gifts to loved ones, with secret messages of affection or desire. The brooches sometimes featured symbols of love and affection, such as a rose, a forget-me-not or sprig of ivy.

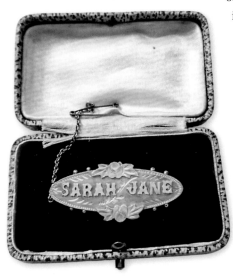

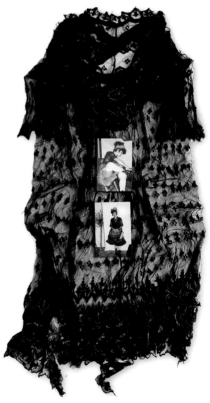

## LOT **134**

### THREE PEN-AND-INK WATERCOLOURS OF SYDNEY SCENES, MID-1980s

$50–$60

Painted by an architect friend, these scenes evoke happy memories of Sydney around the time I first moved here: the vista of the tarmac at the airport, an appropriate place to start; the sweeping curve of Bondi Beach; the harbourside warehouses in Rozelle Bay (pictured here), now long gone to make way for the Anzac Bridge and other massive foreshore scarring. Oh, the parties we had in those warehouses. I had arrived in Sydney and it felt like home.

## LOT **135**

### HAND-STITCHED EDWARDIAN BLACK LACE DRESS (POOR CONDITION), c1910, AND TWO PHOTOGRAPHS, 1986

$10–$20

I acquired this dress at the same time as my beloved jacket (see Lot 70), found in an old trunk in a derelict garage in Sheffield, during my time as a university student. In 1974, the options for dressing 'individually' were few and far between. At boarding school, I had happily spent considerable time practising the reclusive art of creating, stitching and making my own garments. In the thrift stores around Sheffield, I found fabrics from faraway places and clothes from previous generations, and these finds thrilled me to my core.

This dress was so beautiful, so fragile, so ethereal – in a black sort of way. I was experimenting with my dress, mixing things together, occasionally becoming more feminine, yet not overtly sexual or political. As a student of sociology, surrounded by radical thinkers, I found some of their versions of a new world terrifying; yet others made complete sense.

However, hidden in my ambiguous old clothes, my tattered rags, I found an inner security, a comfort zone where I could really explore and discover who I was. The two photographs show me wearing the dress some 12 years after I'd found it, at my 31st birthday party in Balmain, Sydney. By this time, I had my look down. Punk had permitted me to wear black, the stockings are 1920s silks, the pink-net 1950s nylon petticoat had belonged to my mother, and the boots and buckles are described in Lot 136, below.

## LOT 136
### TWO PAIRS OF BOOT STRAPS, TWO PLAITED WOOLLEN STRAPS, AND PHOTOGRAPH, 1986
$10–$20

At a jumble sale in the 1970s, I had found an incredible pair of semi-embroidered, thick black cotton boots with turned-up toes, which I later discovered were Tibetan. I wore them, darned them, wore them and darned them again and again, until eventually they completely disintegrated. The boots had no fasteners, so, to keep them in place, I used woven, plaited or leather straps such as these, wound tightly around my legs. Later, as a punk, I would wear studded stirrups over every form of footwear – even the black gumboots I wore standing in a puddle at Covent Garden market.

The photograph shows me on my 31st birthday, fresh in Sydney, still wearing stirrups over my buckled boots.

## LOT 137
### SIX ITEMS DEPICTING BATS, INCLUDING THREE NETSUKE (JAPANESE MINIATURES), c1920, TWO SILVER CUPS, c1920, AND CARVED STONE PENDANT, DATE UNKNOWN
$450–$550

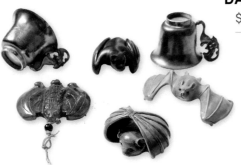

As I had done earlier with the egg-cup collection (Lot 85), now I used the search for bat paraphernalia to open doors to the finest jewellery stores in Australia, including Ben Boulken Pty Ltd. Now long gone, it was owned by the Boulken family and run by two *grande dames*, Esperance and her sister, Madeleine.

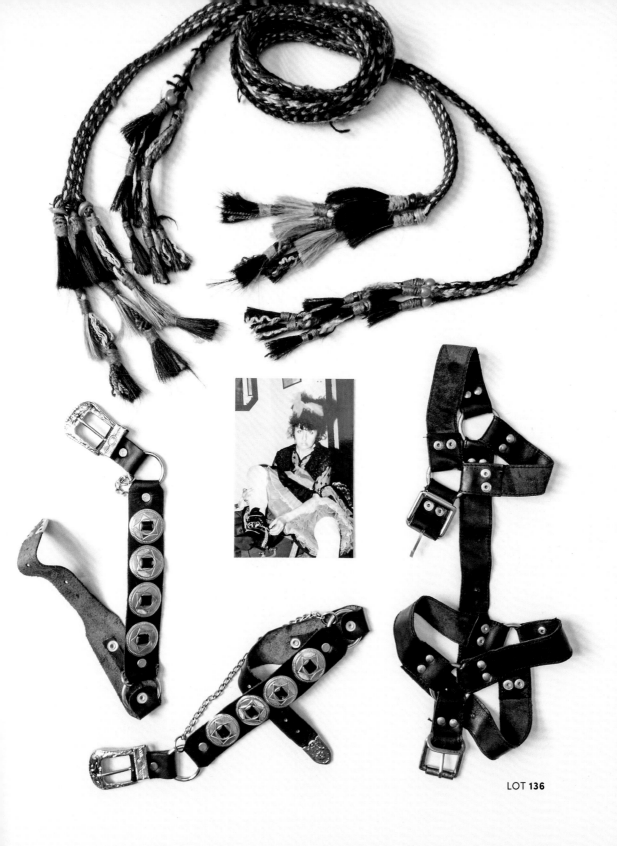

LOT **136**

In the early years when I was making trips between London and Sydney, they became my biggest customers. Back in the day, they would say to me, "We have never known anyone so beautiful try so hard to make themselves look so ugly." No one had ever called me beautiful before. If I ever had to go out with my parents, they would say, "Who'd want to look at you?"

I'm still no good at accepting compliments. The Boulken ladies, however, knew very well what real beauties were hidden in my bag of stock.

LOT **138**

## VICTORIAN BAT'S-HEAD HATPIN WITH GLASS EYES, c1870
$200–$300

Hatpins were worn by women in the West throughout the 1800s and into the 1900s. Their main purpose was to keep hats and veils in place on the head. This was achieved by sticking the steel pin through both the head covering and the hair. These long, sharp pins could also be used in self-defence. In the early 1900s, the number of working women was on the rise. Women were becoming more visible – and being harassed in public. With the advent of the suffragette movement in England and the USA, an item that had been designed for fashion and function was turned into a symbol of resistance. Laws were passed that restricted the length of the pin and required a covering for the 'pointy end'. If you were poor, you had to make do with a piece of potato or cork for the end of your hatpin.

I would love to know something about the woman who wore this hatpin. Was she a 'woman of the night'? Was she in mourning? Was she angry? Was she a 19th-century Goth? Or did she simply have a great sense of humour and a mad look?

LOT **139**

## PAIR OF SILVER EARRINGS SET WITH AMETHYST CABOCHON AND CARNELIAN, BY JOHN PEEBLES
$60–$80

I called these my *Conan the Barbarian* earrings. I bought them in the early 1980s from jeweller John Peebles, who was based just outside Byron Bay, an area I had visited on one of my first trips to Australia.

My daughters remember these as "the earrings Mummy always wore". They were strong, unbreakable and had an air of a warrior woman. Later, as a single parent of twins, they conveyed a message of invincibility, which empowered me and enabled me to face each new day with fortitude and courage.

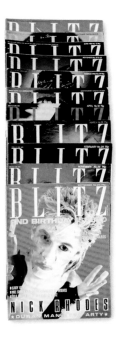

## LOT **140**

### 26 ISSUES OF *THE FACE* AND *BLITZ* MAGAZINES, 1984–1986

$50–$70

In the 1980s, along with antique jewellery, I was bringing magazines, T-shirts, all manner of street culture from England to a ready audience in Australia. Now free and based in Sydney, I was the 'shizit'.

Antenna was a cool new London hairdressing salon situated in a little enclave just off Church Street, Kensington. At the end of one buying trip, with all my stock catalogued for export and a bit of cash left in my pocket, I paid the princely sum of £75 for a full head of black and red hair extensions. My own hair was dyed black, and woven into it the new dreads reached down to my bum. I really thought I looked 'the business'.

On the flight back to Australia, our plane stopped for refuelling in Singapore. It was a late-night transit and we all stumbled off the plane, bleary-eyed and (me particularly) dishevelled, into the transit lounge. Few shops were open, the storekeepers hanging around in groups idly observing the befuddled passengers. As I walked past a pair of stunningly groomed Indian women, both with long, thick, straight, glossy tresses, I heard one of them remark to the other, with a sidelong glance at me, "Horrible hair."

These were the last magazines I bought (unless I was in them).

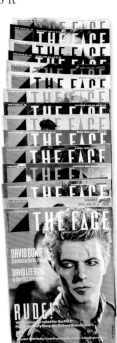

## 'MERMAID' SUITE OF NECKLACE, EARRINGS AND HAIR COMB, 1987, AND 'BRITISH' STOMACHER-INFLUENCED METAL BROOCH BY GREGORY BOLTON, 1987

$150–$250

Soon after I moved to Sydney in 1986, I crossed paths with Gregory Bolton. He was a young, enigmatic and effervescent kid with an incredible eye and a phenomenal knowledge of Egyptian Revival jewellery. We became friends and together spent many hours poring over pieces of jewellery, broken treasures and vintage findings and components that he had somehow managed to track down in the days before the internet.

Gregory would sit at his table in front of his small portable TV, watching *Dynasty*, *Dallas* and *Days of our Lives*, surrounded by dishes and boxes of components, wire, thread and tassels, creating the most incredible pieces of costume jewellery. I remember being appalled at his viewing choices, but realise now that he was possibly finding inspiration in the glamour depicted in these soaps.

He made the Mermaid Suite especially for me, using iridescent abalone shell and crystals and beads in various shades of sea-blue and green. It reminded me of the exotic shells of my childhood (see Lot 19) and became a fluid link to my grandmother.

The 'British' stomacher-influenced brooch was made from a car part. Very punk-chic.

*The 'British' brooch was made from a car part. Very punk-chic.*

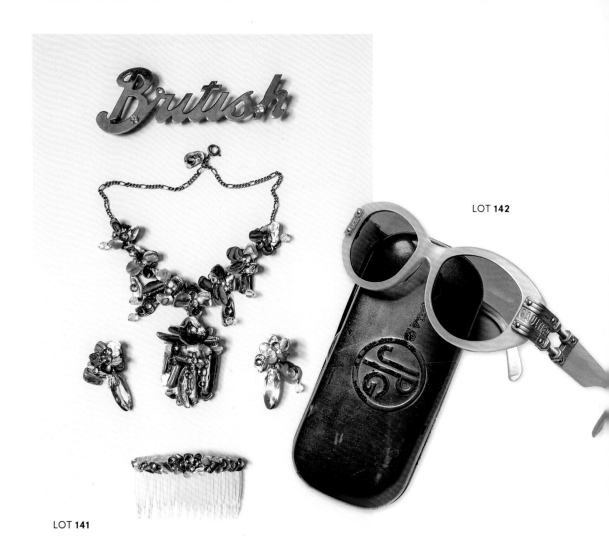

LOT **142**

LOT **141**

LOT **142**

## PAIR OF JEAN-PAUL GAULTIER SUNGLASSES IN ORIGINAL BOX, 1980s

$250–$300

In Australia, 'the lucky country', where the sun shone fiercely for so much of the year, these sunglasses were my go-to accessory. I adored them then and still adore them today. I wore them every single day, come rain or shine. They were tough, resilient and fierce. Behind their dark lenses, I could also feel myself growing into my own power. I, too, was tough, resilient and fierce.

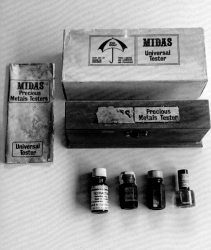
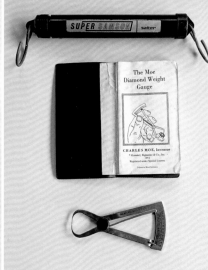
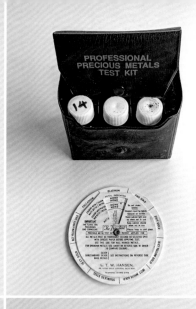
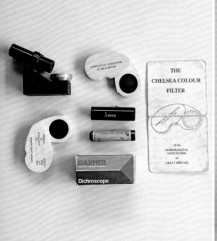
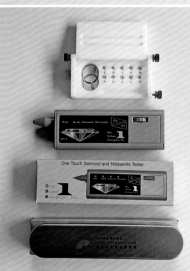
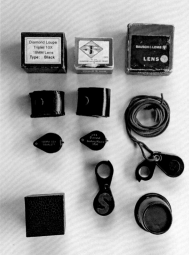
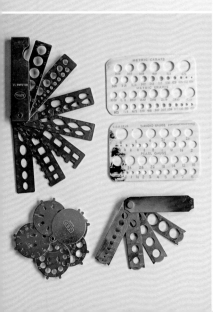
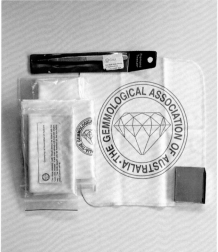
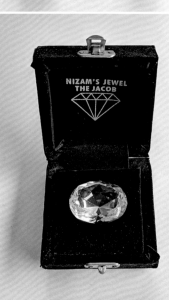

## LOT **143**

### ASSORTED TOOLS FOR JEWELLERY IDENTIFICATION AND TESTING

$250–$300

Tools of the trade. As my business expanded, I started to acquire these for my work: metal-testing acids; diamond gauges; Salter metal scales; loupes; diamond-grading colour master set; diamond testers; Chelsea filter; dichroscope; spectroscope; gem-polishing cloths; tweezers; gemstone profiles and size estimations, to name but a few.

## LOT **144**

### COLLECTION OF ITEMS INCLUDING A SHOE HORN, CHAPATI ROLLING PIN, PARASOL HANDLE AND GLASS SCENT BOTTLE, 1900s AND 1920s

$120–$150

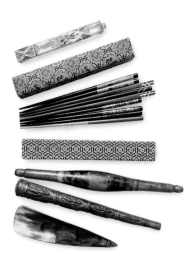

This varied group somewhat represents my varied life over the next few years in Sydney. I was travelling incessantly, mainly between India, England and Australia, and buying and selling all manner of items, including my first property – a house in Newtown. A vibrant, accepting, creative and varied suburb, where I felt comfortable to develop my sense of identity, also reflected in my varied clothing – a reflection of street style that also echoed the subcultures to which I had been exposed.

## LOT **145**

### CHILD'S TRINKET TIN, c1900, CONTAINING FOUR MATCHBOXES, 1987, AND NECKLACE MADE FROM DRIED PIRANHA FISH AND SEEDS, 1987

$40–$60

This small tin makes me so happy. In 1987, I made a trip to South America with an antiques-dealer friend. A life seeking treasures not only included jewels, but also experiences, and this journey was a magical combination of both. We trawled the antiques stores of Buenos Aires, in Argentina, where

I found the tin. The lid cheerfully announces its purpose: *Joyas Para Niños*, which translates as 'Jewels for Children'. What sort of a culture has containers especially made for children to keep their trinkets? Certainly not the one I had come from, where children were expected to be 'seen but not heard'.

We travelled on to Lima, Peru, where I picked up the La Llama matchboxes as a keepsake and purely for their packaging. Finally, we journeyed deep into the Amazon for a week of exploration with local guides. The necklace is the only piranha I kept.

## LOT 146

## 800-GRADE SILVER GAUCHO BELT BY N WOOLLANDS, c1930, NEWSPAPER DATED 2 MARCH 1988, AND PHOTOGRAPH, 1988

$450–$550

The Malvinas (or Falklands) War, was still uppermost in the psyche of the Argentinian people during the time of my visit to Buenos Aires in 1988. These are my two souvenirs from that trip.

Gauchos, the country's traditional stockmen, possess a level of horsemanship, bravery and camaraderie so legendary that they have become a national symbol. I was enthralled to see these gauchos riding the streets. I had never before encountered such men. Their pride, confidence and passionate sense of belonging helped me understand how the Argentinian people must have felt about the British, the foreigners who landed on their territory in 1765, and who eventually took formal ownership of the island territories in 1833.

I bought this central section of a gaucho belt to remind myself of these brave warriors. It is designed as circular-shaped shield, with six flattened sections engraved and decorated with gold-plated flowers. I found it in an *antigüedades* shop in Pasaje de la Defensa, San Telmo, the oldest neighbourhood in Buenos Aires. The central initials (which would have been the original owner's) are A and B. My surname is Adams, and the initial of my travelling companion's surname was B.

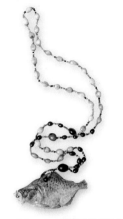

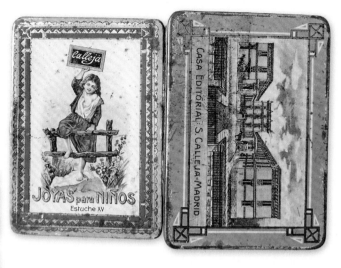

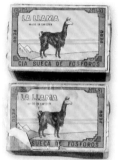

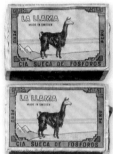

*This small tin makes me so happy.*

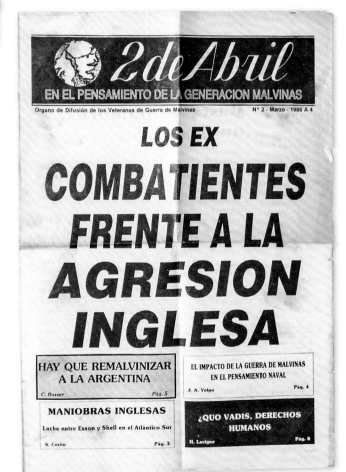

LOT **147**

## COLLECTION OF BAT PARAPHERNALIA

$10–$20

_____

My friends knew I had a fascination with bats, which must have helped them when choosing a gift for someone who, when asked, always answered, "I don't want anything, thank you." The gingerbread bats, too good to eat, were a gift from a gorgeous young woman, Sally Webster, with whom I later studied gemmology, and who has since become a dear friend.

The bat is often associated with spirituality, extra-sensory perception, clairvoyance. My jeweller friend, Gregory Bolton, made me the bat hair comb. He had recently 'inherited' a large tabby cat, Chloe, from a very dear friend who had passed away. Chloe went everywhere with Greg, often draped around his neck, or carried in a tote bag. One day, whilst sitting outside a café far from home, Chloe decided to explore. Despite Greg's searches, the cat could not be found. Greg spent weeks trying to locate Chloe. He offered a reward in newspaper adverts, on local radio and on lamp posts, but no one came forward with information about Chloe.

Eventually, Greg decided to seek help from a psychic. He contacted a woman who lived in the outer suburbs of Sydney and she suggested they meet in a pub that happened to be situated at the top of the street in Newtown where I was now living. Of course, I went along with Greg for moral support and to hear what she had to say.

The psychic and I had never met before; she had no information about me. Unfortunately for Greg, talk of Chloe soon evaporated, as she became focused on her predictions for me. I was going to meet someone from the Middle East – someone with dark, flashing eyes, who spoke a number of languages – and this meeting would change my life. We would meet in the foyer of a grand hotel, and it would have something to do with gold.

I tried to take these forecasts with a pinch of salt. I never stayed in swanky hotels and rarely met gentlemen from the Middle East, but I was quietly troubled by how she could possibly know that I was a jewellery dealer who regularly handled gold pieces.

Within six months of this encounter, at an antiques fair held one Sunday in London's salubrious Park Lane Hotel, I met an Israeli of Iraqi descent, who was to become the father of my twin girls.

Unfortunately, Chloe never returned home to Greg.

And I have never again encountered a clairvoyant.

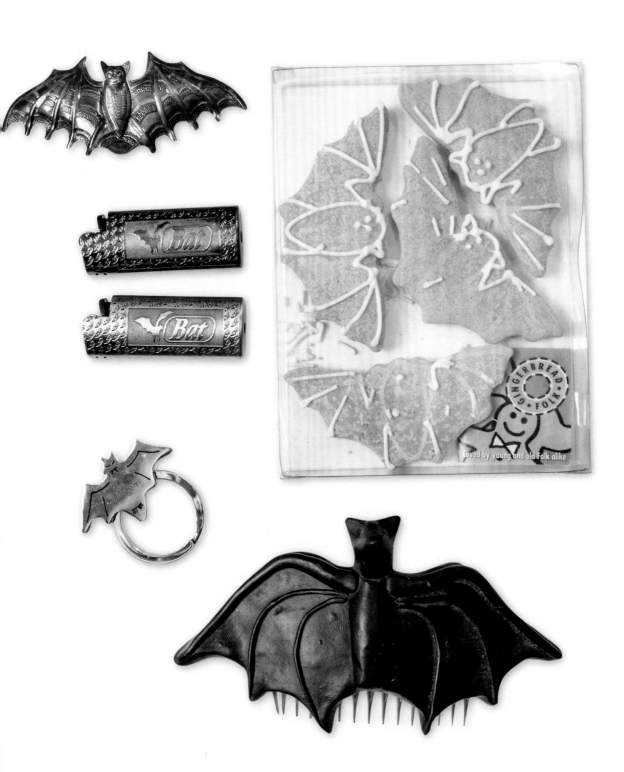

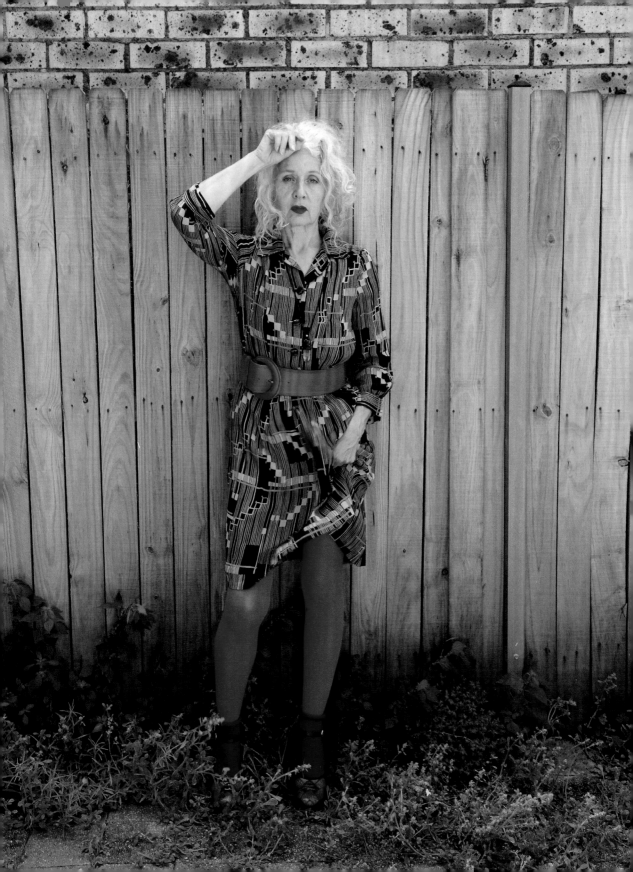

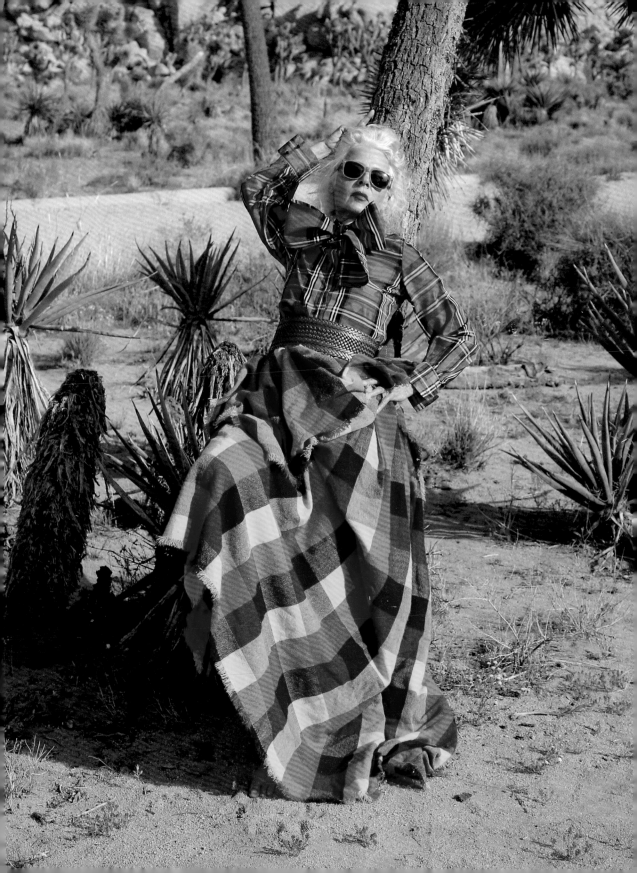

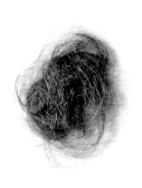

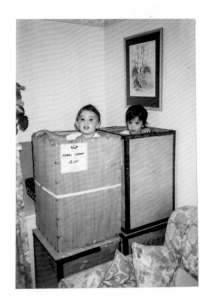

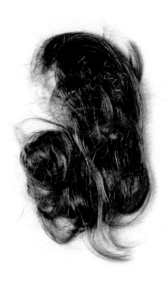

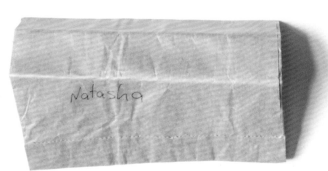

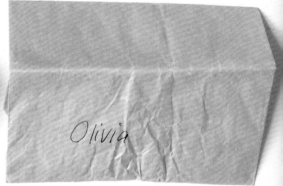

# one long summer

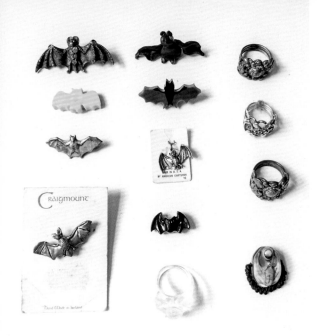

## LOT 148

### COLLECTION OF MINIATURE BAT PARAPHERNALIA, INCLUDING THREE ANTIQUE SILVER CHINESE PUZZLE RINGS, LATE 1800s–EARLY 1900s

$250–$300

The most interesting items here are the three antique Chinese puzzle rings at top right. It is thought that puzzle rings may have originated in China about 2000 years ago, although they are also found in ancient Egypt and the Arabian Peninsula. Legend has it that puzzle rings were invented to monitor a wife's fidelity, as, theoretically, if the ring is removed from the finger, it falls undone. Incidentally, it didn't take me too long to learn the technique of how to put the ring back together.

I acquired these from a dealer friend, who had bought a collection of Chinese antiquities from an elderly lady. The lady had travelled in her youth to what was then a recently independent Tibet. What a woman – what she must have witnessed in her life...

## LOT 149

### COLLECTION OF RETAIL CATALOGUES SHOWING SELECTIONS OF ANTIQUE JEWELLERY STOCK, AND SIX PHOTOGRAPHS, FROM MID-1980s

$1–$5

Through the 1980s and 90s, I was making approximately five to seven trips a year between England and Australia. On each trip I would bring back, on average, 1000 to 1500 handpicked items of antique jewellery. Everything purchased in England had to be more than 100 years old and would be invoiced from my suppliers, catalogued by me, then inspected and subsequently certified as antique by what was known then as the London and Provincial Antique Dealers Association (LAPADA). This was a painstaking process in England, but aided the efficacy of customs clearances and assessment of duties and taxes on arrival in Australia. Speed was of the essence, as I was always planning a quick turn-around for my next buying trip.

The photographs date from the mid-1980s and show me in Australia (and Gaultier), sorting stock into tobacco tins for pricing, prior to showing the new collection to my clients, who would clamour for 'first look'. The bottom five images are a small selection of the silver purchases I made on one trip. There would have been a similar amount of gold pieces, plus many trays of antique rings, as seen in the tobacco tins in the top photograph.

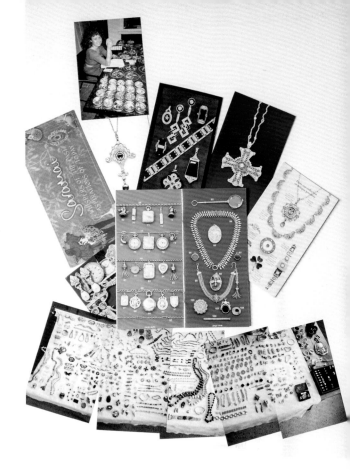

Also shown here is a selection of catalogues, dated from the mid-1980s to 2016, from some of the retailers I supplied. Many of the items in these catalogues were purchased from me.

My father would accuse me of divesting England of its history, whereas I believed that I was a conduit for things to find new homes with people who would become their custodians for another short time.

## LOT 150

## 1970s LEE 101 DENIM JACKET, WITH CUSTOMISED STUDS (SOME MISSING) ON BACK

$20–$40

This jacket has been part of my uniform since the late 1970s. I have no recollection of how it came to me, already worn. It has protected me as a hippie, a punk (I added the skull studs), a street hustler, a traveller, an undercover agent, a hugely pregnant mother-to-be, an invisible, a ratbag and a rebel. It is a garment I feel particularly comfortable wearing. It is the jacket I lived in through the mid-1980s, wearing it with a pair of tatty Levi's

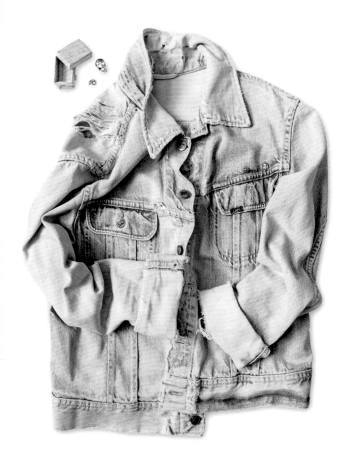

501s, cinched in at the waist with a black leather belt (Lot 111). I would knot the oversized jacket, then do up the bottom button. I had not a care in the world.

Shod in stirrup-decorated cowboy boots, and with plenty of attitude, I would strut my stuff around the globe. Travelling the world, I was independent, unattached and successful, earning a damn good living and doing exactly what I loved. I seemed pleased with myself.

Yet, I knew there had to be more. More. I was living in both Australia and the UK, where I had rented a small basement flat in Shepherd's Bush as my base.

It was at this time, at the age of 33, in the foyer of the Park Lane Hotel in London, that I met the father of my children. We quickly fell for one another. He explained to me that he was married to an English girl for business purposes, which was fine by me, as I had no desire to marry again. He had previously been married to a Canadian (also for business purposes) and seemed accepting of my parallel life and business commitments in Australia.

Only a few months after we'd met in London, we decided to try for a baby. Knowing that a pregnancy so soon into a relationship would be deemed 'unplanned', I confided to my grandmother, Nanny Win, that I was trying to fall pregnant. I simply wanted my critics to know that any child I might be blessed with was wanted, not a 'mistake', and would be loved.

Within a few days of conception, I felt – indeed, I knew – I was pregnant. The scan at six weeks, prior to a solo business trip to Australia, showed two tiny dots.

"Are there twins in your family?" asked the radiographer.

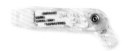

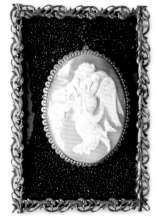

## LOT **151**

### SHELL CAMEO DEPICTING AN ANGEL HOLDING TWO BABIES, c1900, AND THREE PHOTOGRAPHS

$400–$500

I was commuting between London and Sydney, but for citizenship reasons, I chose to give birth in the UK. I carried my twin daughters to full term and they were born either side of midnight in early June 1989, at Queen Charlotte's Hospital, Hammersmith. Gemini twins with different birth dates. It was a 24-hour labour, culminating in a complicated birth. Olivia, my firstborn, weighing 6lb 7oz, needed forceps to be delivered, as by then I was completely exhausted. Tash, at 7lb 6oz, was breech. I counted 25 people in the delivery room, including the twins' excited father. I remember saying, "I feel like I'm on *All Creatures Great and Small*".

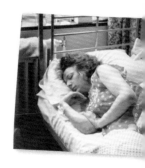

Soon after delivery, I was overcome by the most excruciating pain in my head, far worse than any pain experienced over the previous two days. I remember asking for more gas and air – anything that would alleviate it. I also remember the nurse leaving the room, then nothing.

I awoke two days later. I had suffered two major eclamptic fits and had been unconscious for the first two days of my babies' lives. Drowsy, wired to a drip, which had included the anti-seizure drug Phenytoin, I woke to see Nanny Win worriedly looking at me. My body was now completely covered in a red, itchy, blistering rash – I was allergic to the drug that had probably saved my life. My boobs were as hard as walnuts, completely engorged, as I'd not been able to feed my babies whilst I was unconscious. I remained in hospital for 10 days until I was considered well enough to take my babies home. We were put into a taxi and arrived home to the empty basement flat in Shepherd's Bush.

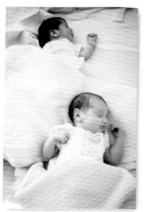

I knew then that I was to become a single parent.

A picture of this brooch features on one of my Instagram posts, dated 11 May 2014, accompanied by the words: *"In the vaults with Saramai. This is one I kept. Remembering those who didn't make it on Mother's Day"* – a reference to my dead twin, and the fragility of life.

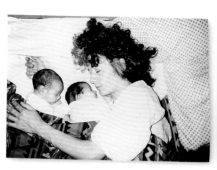

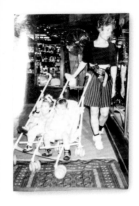

## LOT 152

### BOUCHERON DIAMOND JABOT PIN, IN ORIGINAL BOX, c1980, PAIR OF 18CT GOLD EARRINGS SET WITH A DIAMOND, RUBY AND SAPPHIRE, c1980, PASSPORTS AND PHOTOGRAPHS, 1989

$2000–$2500

The Boucheron pin was a gift from my children's father after their birth. Within two months of their birth, and with English autumn on its way, I'd made applications for the babies' passports. By Christmas 1989, the three of us were living back in my house in Newtown, Sydney. The earrings were the other gift from the twins' father.

Knowing I would be supporting my children alone, back in Sydney, I organised an agent to whom I planned to ship antique jewellery from England. The jewels would be duly processed, authenticated by LAPADA, ticketed, priced and ready to go. My customers were happy with this arrangement, realising that I would be able to source even more unusual items in the London markets if I spent more time there.

## LOT 153

### EIGHT HAND-PAINTED HMSS AND ENAMEL BUTTERFLY BROOCHES, c1900–1940, AND PHOTOGRAPH

$4000–$5000

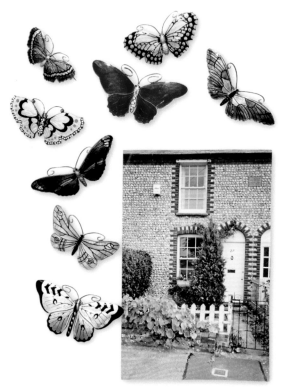

To house us whilst spending the summer months in England, I bought my first UK property, a two-up, two-down Victorian flint cottage in Chichester. It was an idyllic spot overlooking a playground on the outskirts of town. We became a tight little team – the babies seemed to know it was just the three of us, and obliged me by waking up at different times so I could give each of them my full attention. With my babies, I was exhausted but content. We had a routine that became my survival technique. Whenever possible, I ran

LOT **152**

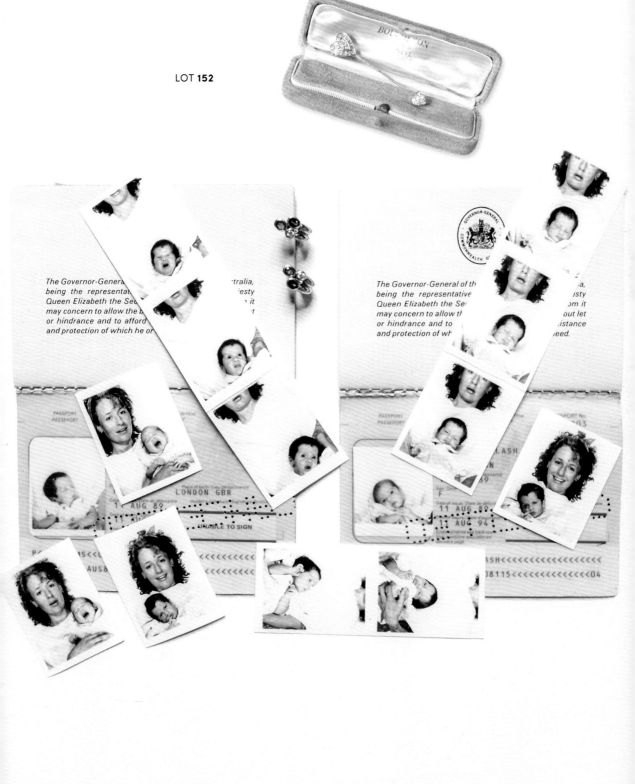

things like a military operation. With an hour and a half between feeds, I would push the double buggy into town, where, with every valuable minute counting, I had to endure intelligent comments such as, "Are they twins?"

## LOT 154
## TWO CUTTINGS OF HAIR WITH A PHOTOGRAPH OF THE TODDLERS IN PACKING CASES, 1990 (SHOWN ON PAGE 178)
$1–$5 (WITHDRAWN)

The first few years of my children's lives were one long summer, the three of us moving between Chichester and Sydney as the seasons changed. In England, the children's father would occasionally come on a Saturday to mind the girls, so that I could get to London to meet with my suppliers. But mainly alone, I would trawl the children around the markets in their huge buggy. I needed to work hard and smart, as I was solely supporting the three of us.

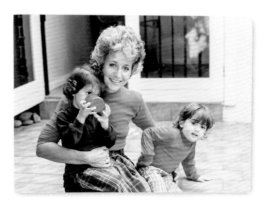

## LOT 155
## TWO HANDMADE COASTERS, AND PHOTOGRAPH, 1991
$1–$5

These lollipop-stick coasters were made for me by my girls when they first started preschool in Glebe, Sydney. Here we are in 1991 – me aged 36, the girls aged two.

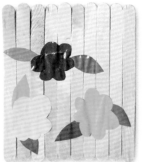
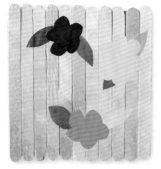

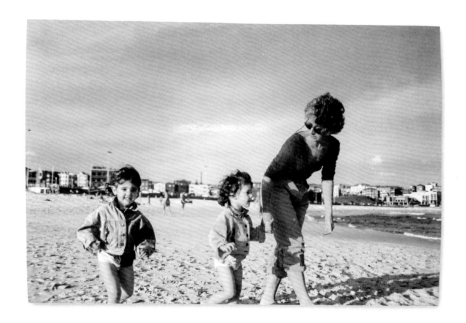

## LOT 156

## LARGE 'BATTLE SHIELD' BROOCH, HMSS, CHESTER, 1891, AND PHOTOGRAPH, SYDNEY, 1991

$750–$1000

I was a warrior, fighting for the three of us. I never asked for assistance with my children and I protected them fiercely. There were troubles with their father, who, despite the fact that we were not together, was coming and going between London, South Africa, Israel and Sydney. This irregularity messed with all our heads, but I gave the girls as stable a life as I could, battening down the hatches when necessary. To all intents and purposes, I believe they had a happy childhood. At age six, the endless summers stopped, as we settled in Sydney to facilitate the children's attendance at the local primary school, where I requested they be placed in separate classes.

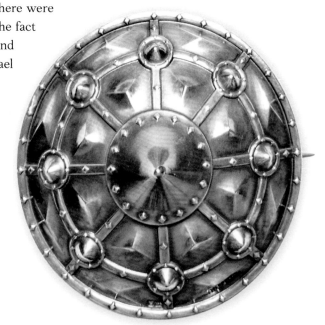

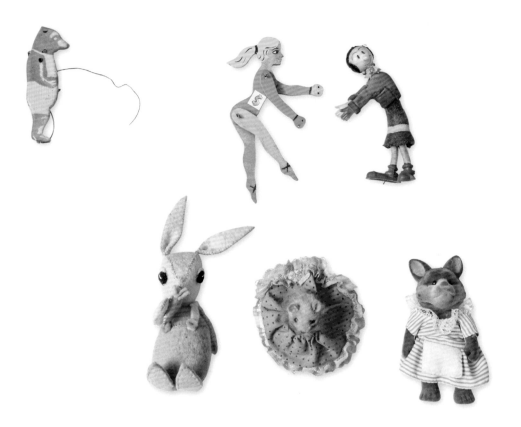

LOT **157**

## COLLECTION OF SIX TOY CHARACTERS, INCLUDING A VICTORIAN MOVING TIN BEAR, OLIVE OYL, c1920, AND JOINTED GYMNAST, 1970s

$120–$150

Juggling roles became the order of the day, starting early to prepare the children for school. They were always neat and clean, with healthy packed lunches. Olivia's long braids would be plaited, and clean school uniforms included (I quote from a schoolteacher) "sensible knickers". I would drop them punctually at school, then take to the road in my sporty red Subaru, visiting my clients who had a voracious appetite for my stock.

Business was booming, my children and I were content, the routine worked and life was good. As we waited to collect our children after school at the end of the day, I was clearly an older mother, working, single and standing apart from most of the younger parents. Although polite, I kept myself to myself – my children, my work and my gay male friends were all I needed to complete my world.

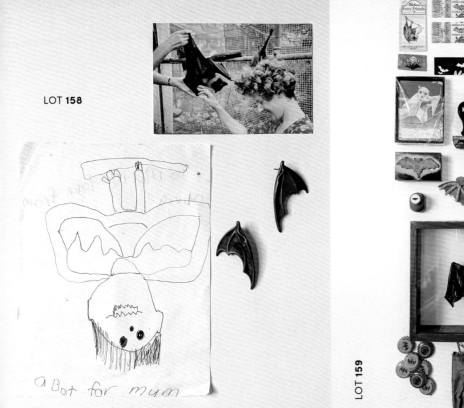

LOT **158**

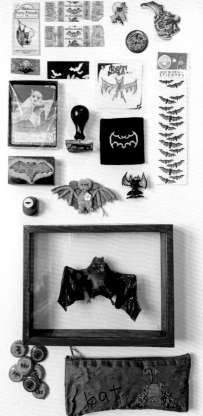

LOT **159**

## LOT **158**

### PAIR OF 'BAT WING' PEWTER EARRINGS, 1980s, PHOTOGRAPH, EARLY 2000s, AND DRAWING, MID-1990s

$5–$10

Young Olivia drew this bat for me; the photograph was taken in a bat sanctuary in Queensland. I never wore the pewter bat earrings, as the children would pull them – or get poked by them. I rarely wear jewellery.

## LOT **159**

### TAXIDERMY BAT IN A GLASS CASE, c1980, WITH AN ASSORTMENT OF BAT-THEMED PARAPHERNALIA

$20–$30

Most of the bats here are made from paper; the pink bat was drawn for me by my daughter, Tash.

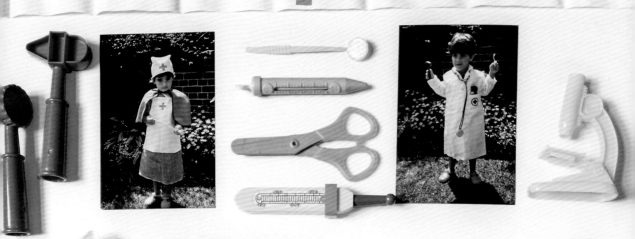

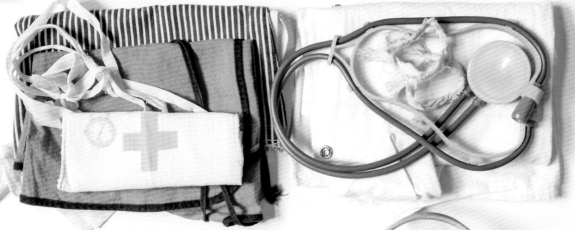

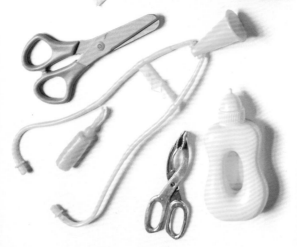

LOT **161**

FIRST AID

BOOTS · NOTTINGHAM · ENGLAND

## LOT **160**

## PONY-SKIN GAUCHO BELT WITH COINS FROM URUGUAY, c1980, LATER CUSTOMISED WITH CHAINS AND KEYS

$30–$40

The gauchos of Argentina and Uruguay traditionally had their belts custom-made with central pieces depicting their family or *estancia* (estate or ranch) name. I found this belt, studded with Argentinian pesos, in a flea market just outside London. I knew immediately how I would customise it.

During Victorian times, it became popular for women to wear a chatelaine – a sort of handbag, if you will. A series of chains, often incredibly elaborate and decorative, that attached to a belt, from which women could hang all their *nécessaires* – needle cases, scissors, dance cards and keys to private and secret places. My chains were tough. No one had access to the old keys, as they were held tightly by me. Locked up tight and hard to open, those chains shouted "Leave me be".

## LOT **161**

## VINTAGE FIRST AID BOX CONTAINING PLASTIC INSTRUMENTS, 1960s, CHILDREN'S DRESS-UP CLOTHING, AND PHOTOGRAPHS, 1990s

$20–$30

The cadet-blue plastic First Aid box is a relic from my childhood camping trips, when preparation of the medicine box was a ritualistic process. We were setting out into unknown territories and needed to be ready to face any emergency. In those days, it was filled with pills for tummy upsets, plasters, calamine lotion and thin gauze bandages.

In the 1990s, on a school holiday trip to the UK, the First Aid box was given a new purpose as the flying-hospital case for Doctor Ollie and Nurse Natasha. Together, using the instruments contained therein, my twin girls carried out many bodily 'explorations' and 'operations'.

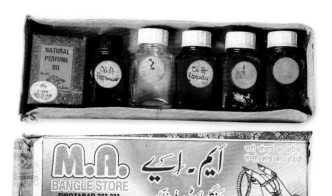

## LOT **162**

### BANGLE BOX CONTAINING SIX NATURAL OILS, c1990s

$20–$30

I purchased these oils in Jaipur, India. Whilst travelling, instead of the traditional Western medicine kit, I would carry these oils as remedies for occasional irritations such as mosquito bites, sinus or throat issues, or muscular pains. These days, I carry nothing medicinal, as everything can be found, pretty much anywhere you travel. Oh, how the world has changed in such an incredibly short time.

## LOT **163**

### SIX DRAWERS FROM A JEWELLER'S BOX CONTAINING TINS, TOOLS AND SPARE PARTS

$200–$300

This miniature chest of drawers contains a mix of spare parts collected over years of trading as a jewellery dealer. No gems; mostly broken items and 'findings' – items useful for restoring antique pieces.

## LOT **164**

### TWO HANDMADE CERAMIC LIDDED BOXES, 1997

$1–$5

In some ways, these years are the lost years. We lose ourselves as we become who others identify us as, who others need us to be. Responsibilities, expectations, demands. These boxes were made for me by my daughters. I have become a grey and pink knob. Accept reward and take joy from the small stuff.

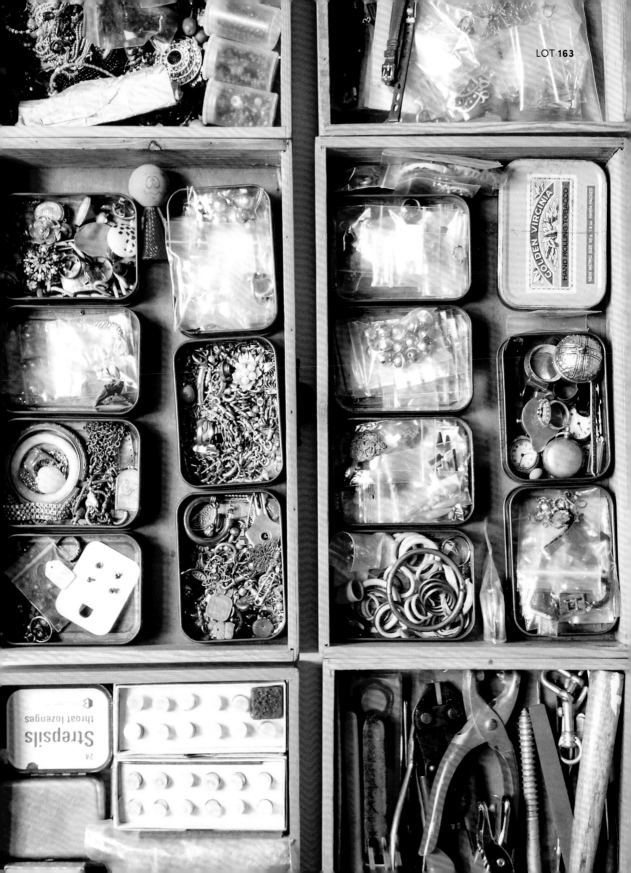

LOT 163

GOLDEN VIRGINIA
HAND ROLLING TOBACCO

Strepsils
throat lozenges
24

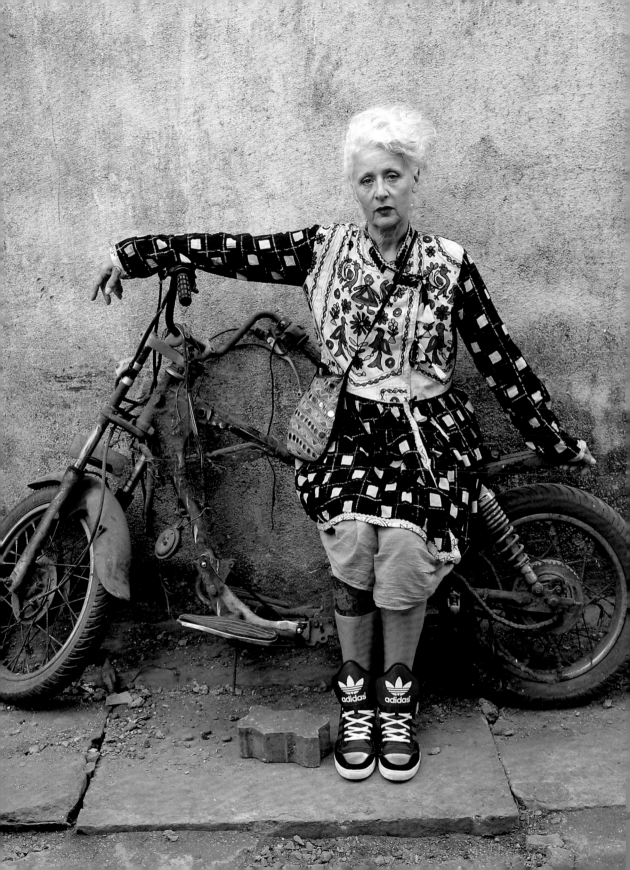

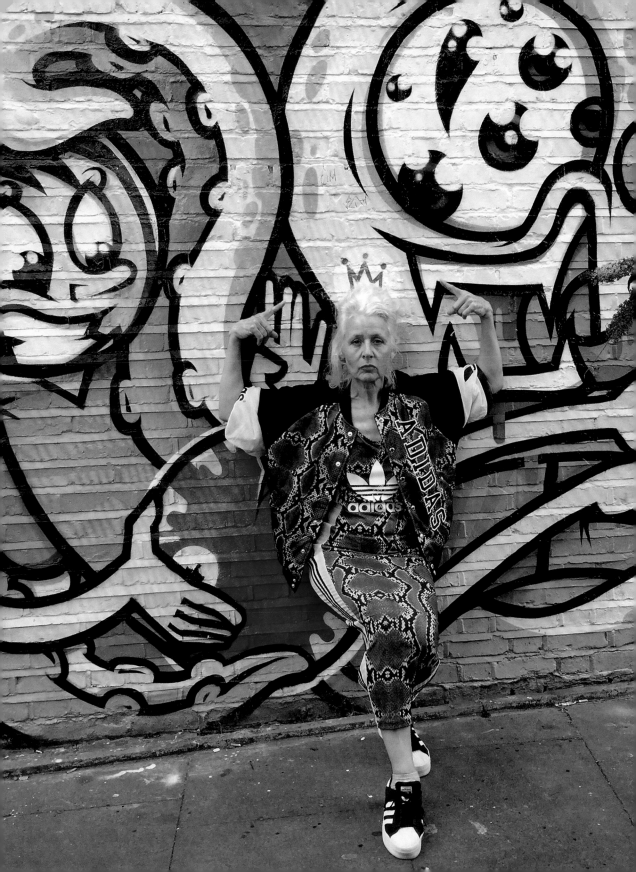

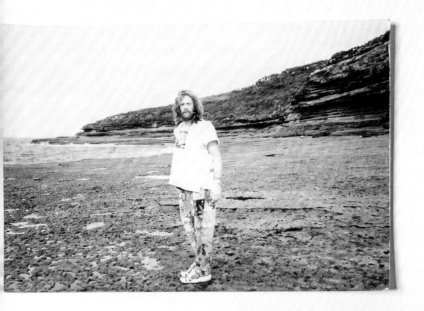

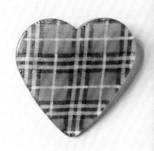

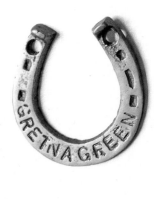

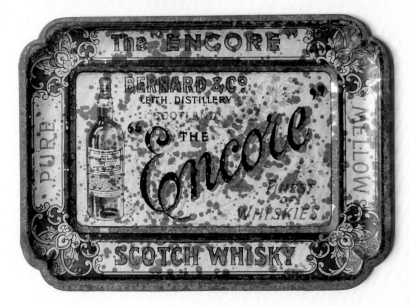

LOT **166**

# CHAPTER 11

# I don't believe in coincidences

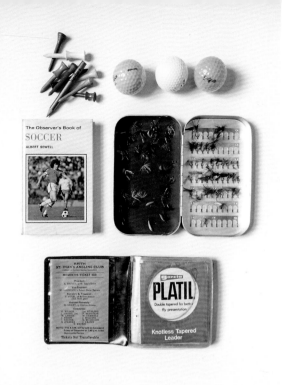

## LOT 165
## A COLLECTION OF FISHING EQUIPMENT AND OTHER PARAPHERNALIA, c1980
$20–$30

A man came into my life through my children's primary school. For some months, a fluid group of people would take the children on outings and it brought me great joy to witness the girls taking part in activities beyond the experiences I could provide. We went camping, bush-walking and fishing – all new pursuits to the three of us. A new normality crept in, one where a strong, dependable and trustworthy male role model quietly had a place.

## LOT 166
## MINIATURE 'THE ENCORE SCOTCH WHISKY' TRAY, c1900, 'GRETNA GREEN' HORSESHOE, c1970, TARTAN HEART, c1980, AND PHOTOGRAPH, 1996
$15–$30

I don't believe in coincidences. In 1996, when my girls were seven, circumstances pushed this man and me together. The way we found one another was complicated, somewhat guided by 'frenemies' and, despite attempts at resistance, a slow and unexpected force completely overtook us. Our long-developing friendship exploded into an inferno, as misunderstandings and rumours fuelled a smouldering fire and we joined forces. Both solitary beings and not influenced by others' opinions, this 'Big Man' and I acknowledged that we had each found our other.

## LOT **167**

## DRAWING-PIN TIN CONTAINING VARIOUS UNSET CAMEOS, THREE HARDSTONE CAMEOS, c1900, AND JAN LOGAN JEWELLERY CATALOGUE, 1999

$900–$1200

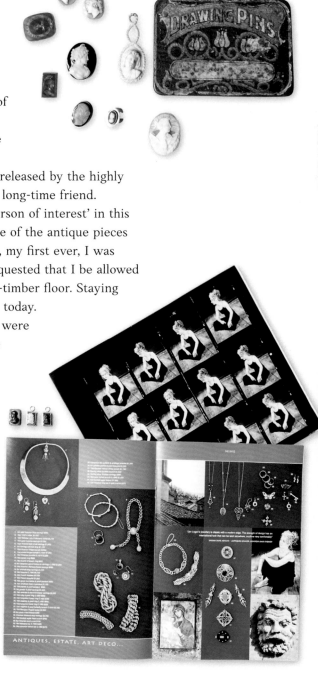

I gathered these individual miniature works of art to use in repairs or remakes. Sometimes, unexpectedly, a mismatched pair would unite – a bit like life, really.

The jewellery catalogue is one of the first released by the highly successful jeweller, Jan Logan, my client and long-time friend. In 1999, Jan asked me to be featured as a 'person of interest' in this catalogue, which also contains images of some of the antique pieces I had supplied to her store. During the shoot, my first ever, I was uncomfortable standing around posing, so requested that I be allowed to remove my shoes and sit on the old rough-timber floor. Staying grounded worked for me then, as it still does today.

The hardstone cameos, in reverse colours, were my twist on Jan's concept of interchangeable drop earrings.

*Sometimes, unexpectedly, a mismatched pair would unite – a bit like life, really.*

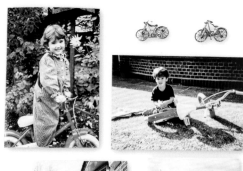

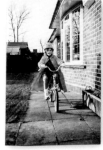

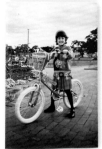

## PAIR OF HANDMADE 15CT GOLD 'BICYCLE' BROOCHES WITH MOVING PARTS, c1900, AND FOUR PHOTOGRAPHS, VARIOUS DATES

$3000–$3500

For their seventh birthday, I bought each of the children a new pink bicycle. Meanwhile, the Big Man had been locked out of his home, his few possessions left on the pavement. He was forced to hurriedly rent a place, having effectively being told, "On yer bike!"

The bicycles remained hidden for two weeks prior to the girls' birthdays, taking up most of the floor space in his tiny apartment. Natasha is seen with her bike in the bottom-right photo, wearing the jumper in Lot 173.

I purchased the perfect miniature gold bicycle brooches soon afterwards on our inaugural trip together to India.

## SILVER PENDANT OF AN ORANGE ENAMELLED SUN, ON LEATHER STRAP, c1970, AND PHOTOGRAPH, 1998

$30–$40

I am the eternal optimist. Energy from the sun – fire – forms the core of my being. One overcast day in the late 1970s, I found this wonderfully exuberant enamel pendant, which represents optimism, hope, rejuvenation and life itself. The Big Man wears it in this photograph. Everywhere, we were being tested. At a teacher's request, the children had to be moved to a different school. Although the girls were in no way responsible for my actions, I conceded in order to protect them. Many people in my neighbourhood, Newtown, had stopped speaking to me. The forces that could have broken the Big Man and me apart were, instead, solidifying our commitment, filling us with resilience and strength.

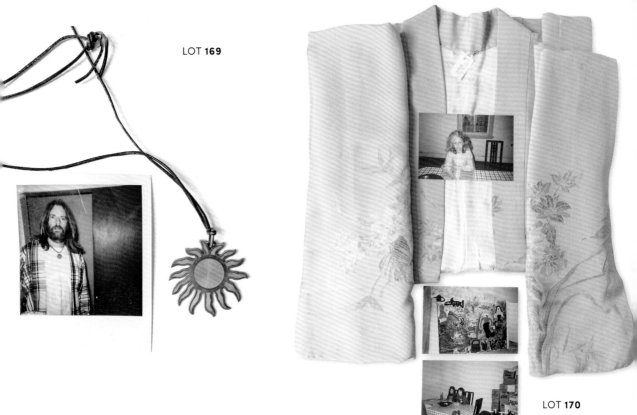

LOT **169**

LOT **170**

LOT **170**
## VINTAGE PINK SILK KIMONO, c1940,
## AND THREE PHOTOGRAPHS, 1996
$20–$40

For seven years I had been a contented, hardworking and well-functioning single parent to my two girls. However, in 1996, my 41st year, major life upheaval was happening on all fronts. A letterbox-drop alerted me to the forthcoming auction of a massive, virtually derelict 'grand old lady' – one of the largest terraces in Newtown and only two streets away. I spontaneously viewed it on the Saturday, telling the children to go and "choose their bedrooms", hand-delivered a contract to my wonderful solicitor on Sunday, made a cheeky offer prior to auction on Monday and exchanged on Tuesday. I requested a lengthy settlement period, because, although my business was booming, being a single, self-employed woman made it tricky for me to get a mortgage. I needed to sell my now-unencumbered first home to pay outright for this property. Yep – I've always taken risks, but they were calculated and I was confident that it would happen.

This major shift was occurring at the same time as the shift in my personal life – challenging waters to navigate.

After many months of upheaval, during which I reached into the depths of my being for strength, I actually found it in the Big Man, who had quietly and gently become my rock. When the time came to move into my massive dump of a mansion, we moved in together.

Within a month, I collapsed with pneumonia and was severely ill for the next six months. Finally, with a dependable human by my side, I could let go. The photos are taken at this time.

I had become known in the neighbourhood as 'The Pink Lady', because I frequently wore pink. Some years later, when the Big Man and I started a secondary jewellery business, it seemed only fitting that the brand colour be a dirty pink.

LOT **171**
## BRONZE MINIATURE LADDER, c1900, AND COLLECTION OF 9CT GOLD LADDER CHARMS, c1930
$70–$100

For the first time in my life, I had a true partner. We understood one another. We had one another's backs and discussed absolutely everything

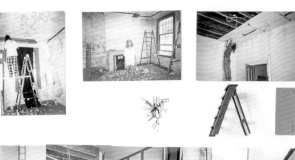

honestly and openly. Acknowledging that the change of circumstances had been tricky for the children, we focused mainly on their wellbeing. When he wasn't out on other jobs, the Big Man worked tirelessly on the house. My enduring image of him is up a ladder, hence these items. Both of us had had solitary jobs, so we recognised the need for alone time – the time to do our own thing, fully trusting the other's loyalty and fortitude. I combined working at an auction house with making short trips to London, seeking out original and unusual pieces for my clients. We were juggling life, roles, tasks and skills. We were a great team and life was good.

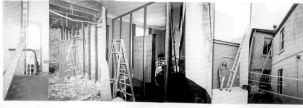

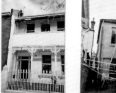

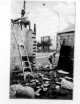

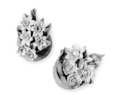

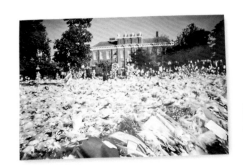

## LOT **172**

**TWO MINIATURE CERAMIC POTS OF LILIES, 1997, AND TWO PHOTOGRAPHS, 1997**

$1–$5

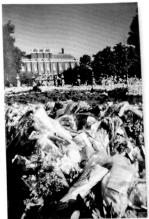

There are events that occur, with which we have no tangible connection, yet we can remember vividly where we were at the time, what we were doing and with whom. One such day was 31 August 1997 – the day Princess Diana was involved in a fatal car accident in a tunnel in Paris.

I was preparing to fly to London on a business trip, where I had by then purchased an apartment in Surbiton.

Diana's funeral was held on Saturday 6 September 1997. I had arrived in London on the previous Thursday, timing it so I could source stock at Portobello Road on the Saturday. I planned to pay my respects to Diana at Kensington Palace, where I arrived before dawn to find the lawns completely covered with flowers, candles and countless groups of people huddled together, clearly shocked and devastated. It was an outpouring of grief the like of which I had never witnessed before nor since.

I remained at Kensington Palace for many hours, wandering amongst the throngs and strolling along the side of the palace, where there were fewer people. From a distance, I quietly observed movements around the gun carriage that would carry her to Westminster Abbey. It seemed such a solitary, private moment – one captured in my mind's eye that will remain with me forever. Diana's coffin was covered with white lilies. Pure, chaste white lilies – majestic flowers associated with the Virgin Mary, Queen of the Angels.

I bought these little pots of lilies later the same day.

*I arrived before dawn to find the lawns completely covered with flowers, candles and countless groups of people...*

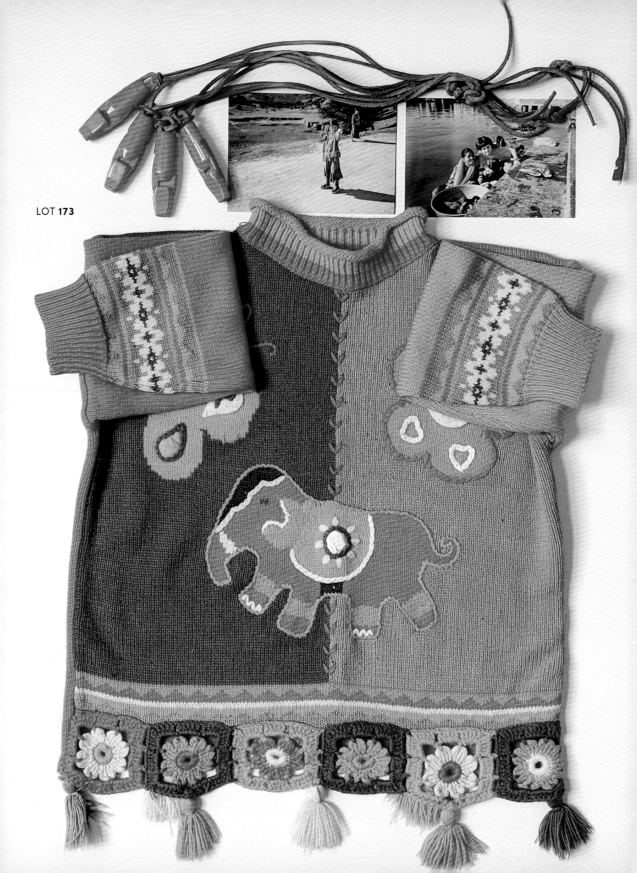

LOT **173**

## LOT **173**

## CHILD'S JUMPER, FOUR RED WHISTLES ON LEATHER STRAPS, AND TWO PHOTOGRAPHS, ALL 1997

$10–$20

We travelled to India for the first time as a family when the children were seven. Each of us was armed with a bright red, really loud plastic whistle. We wore them at all times when we were out and about. The children had clear instructions that, should we become separated, they must blow their whistles and we would come and find them. The whistles remain unblown.

## LOT **174**

## VINTAGE SILK AND SILVER-THREAD SARI, DATE UNKNOWN, SELECTION OF INDIAN COSTUME JEWELLERY, 1997, AND TWO PHOTOGRAPHS, 1997

$50–$80

In 1997, on my father's birthday, 29 December, the Big Man and I were married in Jaipur, in an intimate ceremony of just the four of us. Our marriage, a traditional Hindu ceremony, was performed by the senior Pandit of Jaipur under a canopy of marigold garlands, with our girls close by.

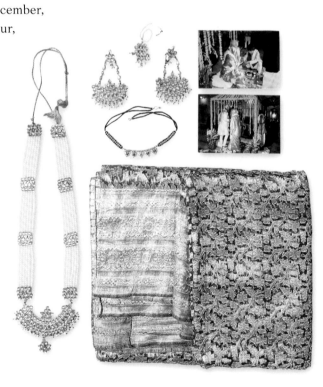

My beautiful second-hand sari was purchased three days prior to the ceremony from a nomadic woman trader in the sprawling bazaar just outside the city walls of Jodhpur.

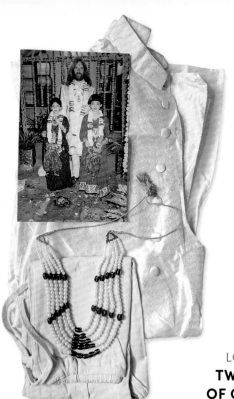

## LOT 175

### CREAM BROCADE SHERWANI AND COTTON SHALWARS, ASSORTED COSTUME JEWELLERY AND PHOTOGRAPH, ALL 1997

$20–$30

Big Man's wedding suitings includes the Indian version of a knee-length fitted frock coat (sherwani), with baggy cotton trousers (shalwars). His costume jewels fittingly came from the street markets of Jaipur, purchased the day before our wedding.

## LOT 176

### TWO DRAWERS CONTAINING BOXES OF GLASS AND PLASTIC INDIAN BANGLES, 1980s–1990s

$40–$60

The red, golden and white boxed set of bangles are the ones I wore at my wedding. They are plastic imitations of the traditional Punjabi chooda (or choora), ivory and red bangles, the red signifying energy and prosperity. I wore mine for a few days, although, traditionally they are worn for a minimum of 40 days after the ceremony. After marriage, Indian custom requires a woman to wear bangles to signify the long life of her husband. Different-coloured bangles represent different wishes, and traditions vary from state to state. In Maharashtra, western India, for example, the bride wears an odd number of green glass bangles, representing new life and creativity. In Tamil Nadu to the south, wearing green glass bangles alongside gold ones signifies prosperity and fertility.

*After marriage, Indian custom requires a woman to wear bangles to signify the long life of her husband.*

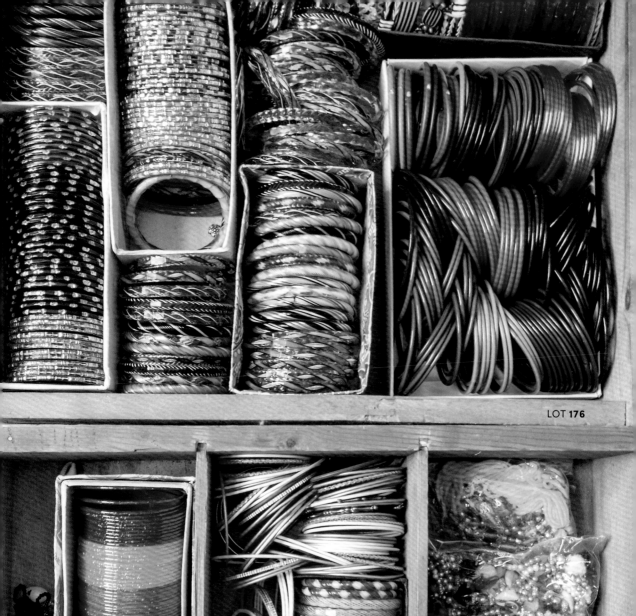

LOT 176

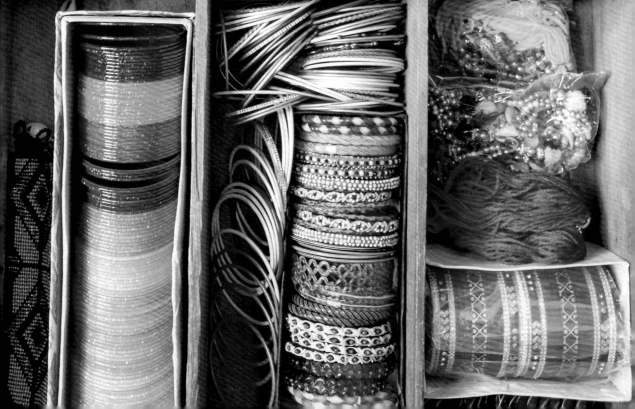

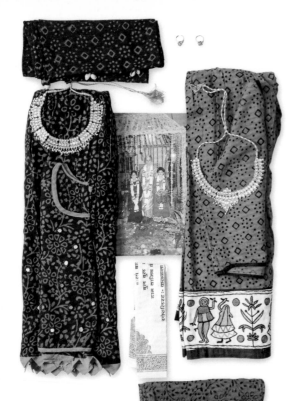

## LOT 177

### TWO TRADITIONAL RAJASTHANI GIRLS' DRESS SETS AND PHOTOGRAPH, ALL 1997

$20–$40

The outfits worn by my girls for the marriage ceremony in Jaipur – simple, understated and comfortable. It was a private ceremony and the beautiful garlands and costume trinkets were decoration enough for my girls during this intensely precious celebration.

## LOT 178

### SILK DUPATTA (SCARF), GREEN SILK EVENING GOWN MADE FROM VINTAGE SARI, AND PHOTOGRAPHS

$50–$100

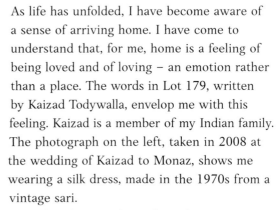

As life has unfolded, I have become aware of a sense of arriving home. I have come to understand that, for me, home is a feeling of being loved and of loving – an emotion rather than a place. The words in Lot 179, written by Kaizad Todywalla, envelop me with this feeling. Kaizad is a member of my Indian family. The photograph on the left, taken in 2008 at the wedding of Kaizad to Monaz, shows me wearing a silk dress, made in the 1970s from a vintage sari.

In the photograph on the right, I'm wearing a scarf on my wrist. It came from my grandmother and is covering some of the enamel bangles, which I'd just purchased in one of the main stores (Lot 230). The photograph shows me ordering the 'Saramai' seals, seen in Lot 218.

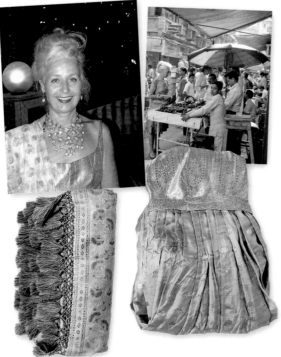

## LOT 179
## COLLECTION OF ORIGINAL HANDPAINTED ART DECO JEWELLERY DESIGNS, c1930
$350–$450

These finely detailed original watercolours are handpainted designs of jewels, mainly earrings, created for P. Dubash & Co, a jeweller once situated in Bombay (Mumbai). The entire collection was a gift to me from my Parsi Indian family and I treasure them for so many reasons.

The words that follow are written by Kaizad Todywalla:

*"I first met Sarah when I was a teenager and she and my father were doing business together. Years later, when Sarah and David were married, they became honorary Todywallas, indispensable family members through good times and bad. We forgot that we were unrelated and hailed from different and very diverse beginnings, and now Sarah is a confidante to my mother and aunts, and also an objective sounding board to us kids. One day I anointed Sarah with the title 'Saramai' — 'mai' meaning mother, a term of endearment and respect. I also renamed David as 'Big Man Taylor' in reference to his large frame, big feet and broad smile! It was a matter of great pride and joy when Sarah chose the name Saramai for her jewellery brand; this confirmed how much our lives are entwined.*

*When, quite by chance, Saramai exploded on the Internet, we had to share our Saramai with a world of people. Strangers loved her, followed her, smitten by her fierce spirit. People were forced to open their eyes and look beyond the glam, glitter and plastic to look into the spirit and soul of a person who*

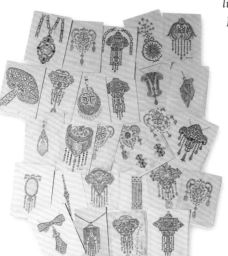

*literally just wore her inner self on her sleeve. Here is this beautiful woman who wears her lines proudly, for they show the world endless stories of her tumult and her success, her strife and her joys, her dreams and her aspirations, some fulfilled, some yet to be and some that may never be. Over the years we have shared our joys and our travails, and somewhere in this journey spanning decades our lives intertwined such that today we are but one family even though oceans may separate us."*

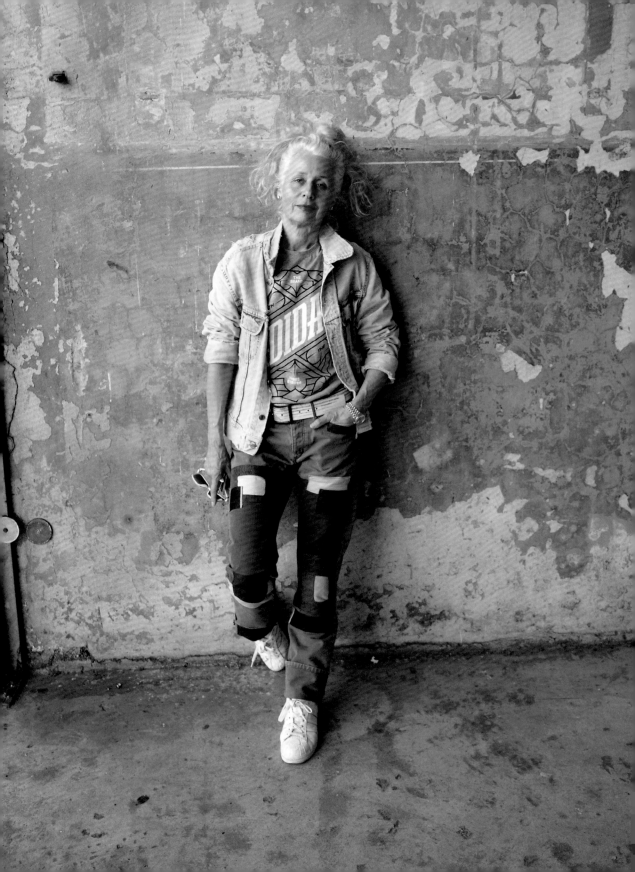

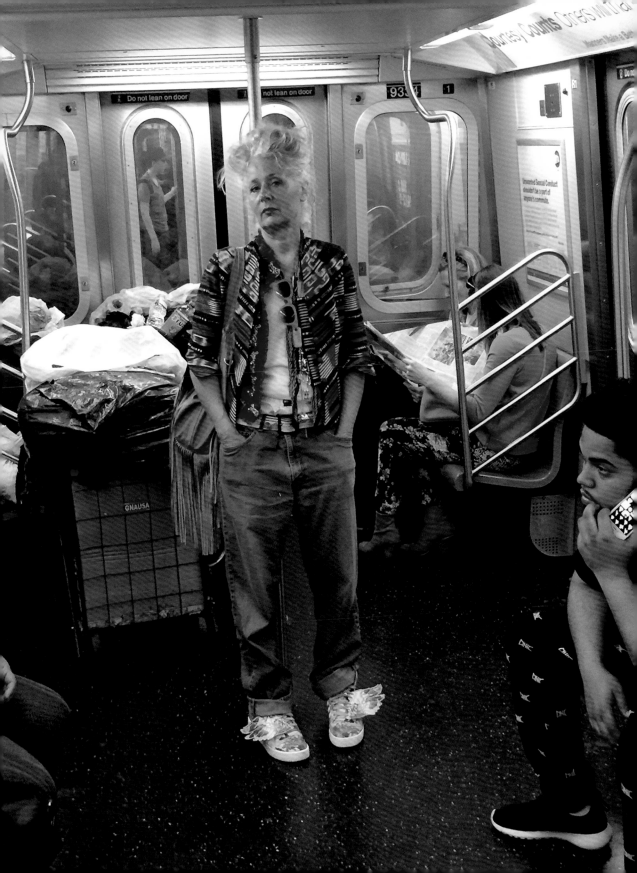

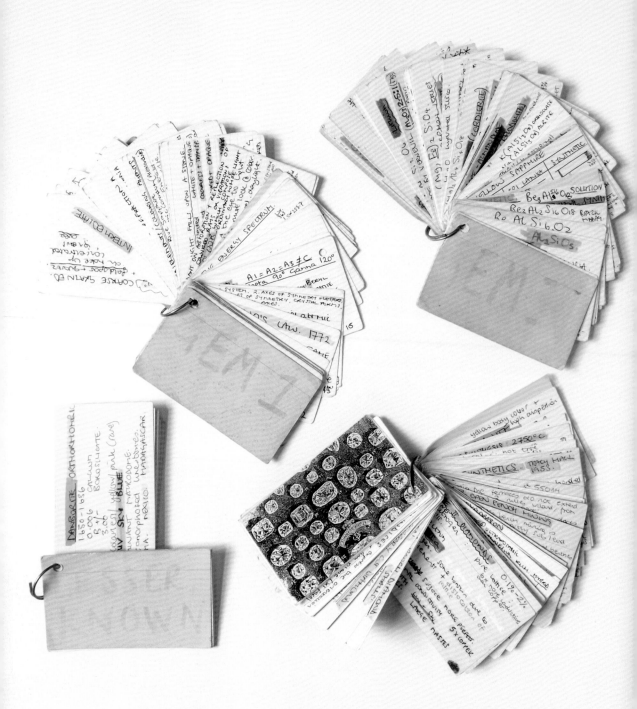

LOT **183**

# crossing boundaries

## LOT **180**

### ASSORTED PHOTOGRAPH ALBUMS DOCUMENTING HOUSE RENOVATIONS, 1996–2000 (NOT SHOWN)

$5–$10

Base Camp for the next 20 years became our huge, 1870s Victorian terrace house in Newtown. Together, the Big Man and I restored the entire property. We had the vision and the time, the passion and the knowledge, the understanding and the love. Over many years, our skills produced an incredible home, and our happiest times were when we were creating it.

## LOT **181**

### GEORGIAN 15CT GOLD RING WITH HANDPAINTED MINIATURE DEPICTING A YOUNG GIRL, c1820, AND PHOTOGRAPH, 2008

$1800–$2000

Prior to the invention of photography, the wealthy would commission artists to paint their loved ones. This portrait of a child in Regency dress is painted on ivory and set under glass. It gives the sense of a childhood in stark contrast to that of my two children, photographed aged nine, nearly 200 years later. On her ninth birthday, the Big Man had taken Tash to have the red streaks put in her hair. It was their very big secret, though little did she know that Big Man and I had discussed it in minute detail.

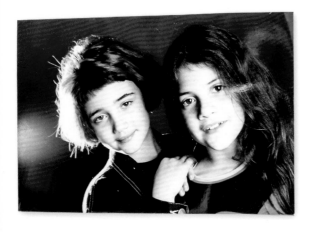

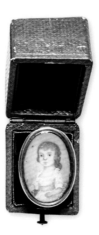

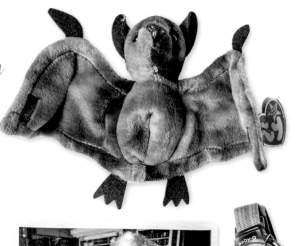

*When I was travelling and away from the children, this was the subject of numerous photographs.*

## LOT **182**

### CASIO BABY-G WRISTWATCH, PLUSH BABY BAT SOFT TOY, AND PHOTOGRAPH, 1990s

$20–$30

The watch and soft toy were two of my travel essentials through the 1990s. The green Baby-G wristwatch was functional and strong, cool and dependable. Equally as important was the baby bat toy. When I was travelling away from the children, it was the subject of numerous photographs. In this one, taken in India, it is nestled amongst a litter of kittens.

## LOT **183**

### FOUR SETS OF CUE CARDS FOR MY DIPLOMA IN GEMMOLOGY, 1998

$5–$10

Cue cards have been my go-to study system since I attended high school. Thanks to the Big Man's support, at the age of 43, I had time to return to study gemmology and quickly fell back into the method. I would summarise, research and add to each lecture. Information would be colour-coded for ease of identification, a shorthand system of retaining a lot of information. It was in the days before mobile phones, before we wasted so much of our time mindlessly scrolling through pulp fiction, and one or other of these babies was permanently in my bag. I did well.

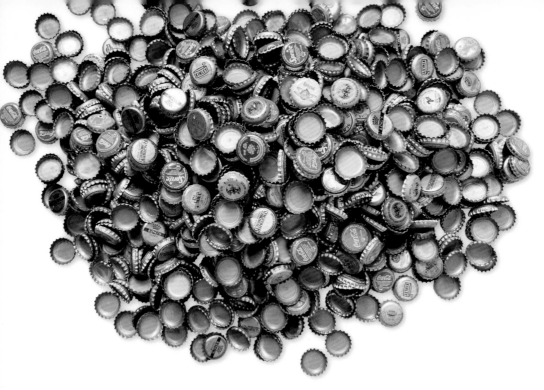

LOT **184**

## COLLECTION OF INDIAN METAL BOTTLE CAPS, 1999

$10–$20

Gathered by my children during a family trip on Palolem Beach, in Goa, southern India.

LOT **185**

## FOUR FULL-SIZE RECORDERS, INCLUDING AN ADLER, BOXED, AND TWO MINIATURES, WITH BOX, 1995

$40–$70

Recorder lessons seem to be a painful rite of passage for children with eager parents. Sheepishly, I have to admit to being one such parent. I'm not sure why, generation after generation, we continue to fall into this trap, as the shrill sound of a painfully disinterested child blowing a recorder has to be as big a punishment for the parent as it is for the child.

My recorder, together with oil, cleaning brush and lengthy instructions (all in German, although, really, how much instruction is needed?), lies in its original neatly labelled box. My daughters' instruments are Bakelite versions, badly labelled with white-out, sans box.

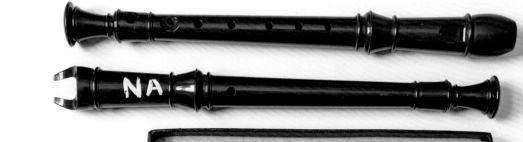

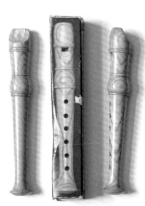

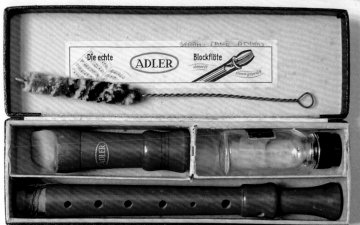

ADLER

Die echte ADLER Blockflöte doppelt steam-gespült

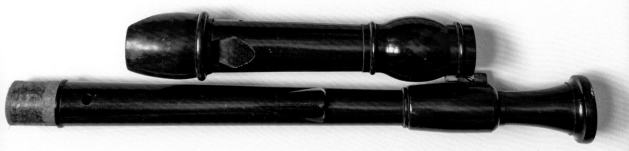

lot 185

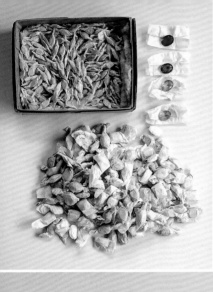
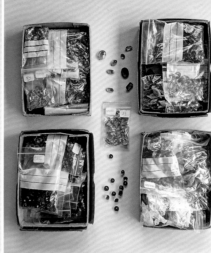
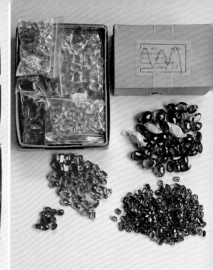
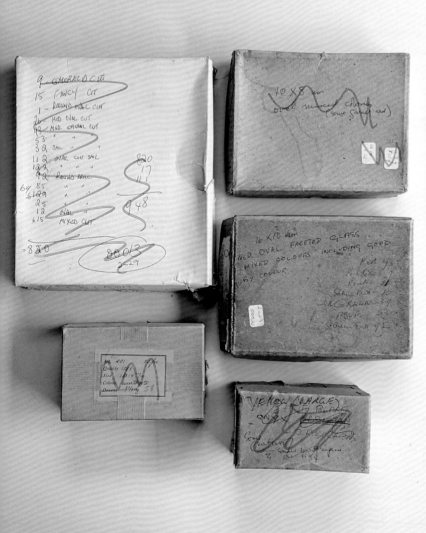
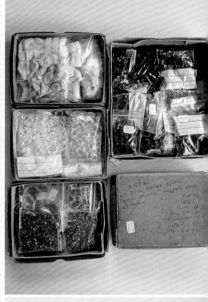
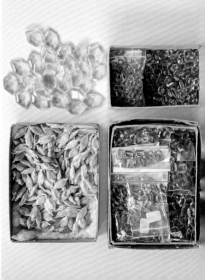

# BOX OF VARIOUSLY COLOURED PASTE GEMSTONES, c1920

$400–$600

The gemmology course, undertaken over a number of years, was a way of formalising, expanding and deepening my knowledge of the gemstone component in jewellery. One weekend, the gemmology department was having a major reshuffle of the labs and redistributing the contents of the library, so a few of us 'gemmos' volunteered to help.

This box of coloured glass stones was found deep in the recesses of a cupboard at the top of the building, a room where random stuff had gathered and long been forgotten. In the rarefied world of gemstones, these fake, colourful and brash imitations of the 'real thing' were considered unworthy. I, however, was completely entranced, mainly, I admit, by the way each one had been individually and lovingly wrapped in soft, ivory-coloured tissue paper to prevent abrasion of the comparatively soft glass. I was able to buy the entire collection for a song.

Things hold different values for different people. My work as an antiques dealer has been facilitated by recognising this – sensing a certain 'something' in a piece that ensures it will be appreciated and valued in different ways. The gift of recognising an item's appeal, trusting my instinct and having the courage to act on it has helped make me who I am.

These cheerful, brash glass imitators speak of an optimism that rivals their more serious counterparts – those gemstones locked away in safes, too valuable to be given such freedom.

Weirdly though, should these beauties be used to make jewellery, they would immediately lose their appeal to me. Maybe I'm attracted to the fact that they resemble boiled sweets in their individual wrappings.

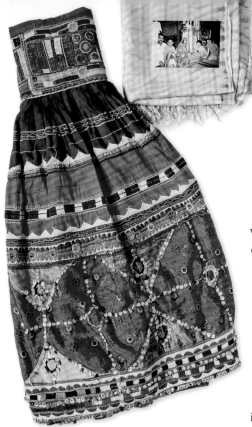

## LOT **187**

### RAJASTHANI SKIRT, DATE UNKNOWN, PINK SARONG, c1980, AND PHOTOGRAPH, 2002

$50–$80

This heavy, vibrantly coloured skirt was made by the woman seen in the photograph, who combined pieces of traditional fabrics and embroidery from various parts of India. Although she comes from the south of the subcontinent, we met on the western beaches of Goa, where she had travelled for business, and is pictured here wearing a similar skirt.

I have been fortunate enough to have spent a considerable part of my life crossing boundaries. I have learnt to adapt to different ways of life, traditions and subcultures, which, in turn, have influenced my personal style of clothing and adornment. Clothes take on different meanings in different contexts. 'Appropriation' has been integrated with respect and reverence to become a part of my life and my dress, and also adopted occasionally to blend in with those around me.

The pink sarong has been with me since the glittery days of the 1980s and is seen here worn by my daughter, Natasha (aka Tash), aged 13.

## LOT **188**

### PAIR OF HANDMADE TIMBER COCKATOO FIGURES, c1970, THREE PHOTOGRAPHS, AND OTHER EPHEMERA, 2000s

$20–$30

Business was going well. As a wholesaler, my overheads were low. I had no need to impress or woo clients by throwing extravagant parties, and I was definitely not a shopper, rarely buying new garments. My wardrobe held clothes I loved, which suited my every purpose.

I decided to purchase an investment property with a view to opening a jewellery shop potentially "in my retirement". So, here is the place. It had been running for some time as Alex Cordobes' iconic pizza shop, adjoining

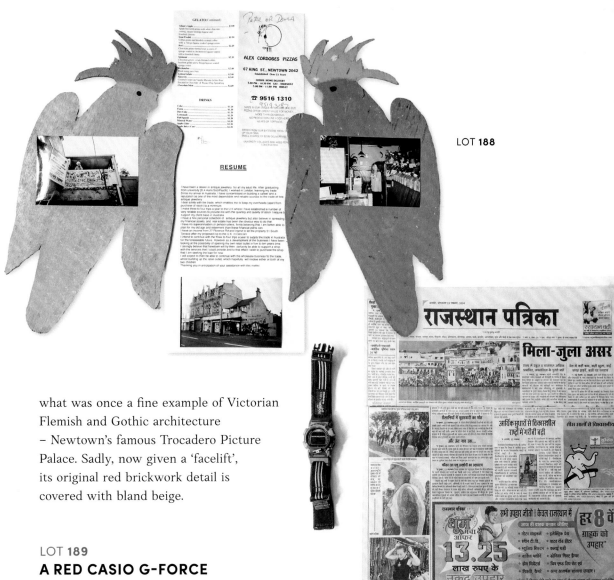

what was once a fine example of Victorian Flemish and Gothic architecture – Newtown's famous Trocadero Picture Palace. Sadly, now given a 'facelift', its original red brickwork detail is covered with bland beige.

## LOT 189

### A RED CASIO G-FORCE GENTLEMAN'S WRISTWATCH, AND INDIAN NEWSPAPER, 2004

$30–$40

Matchie-matchie on our travels in our G-Force wristwatches. The newspaper features a rare sighting of the Big Man. This photo was taken on a family holiday in Mahabalipuram, Tamil Nadu, where we were attending a dance festival. The Ganesh tatoo, his stature, colouring and (through Indian eyes) likeness to WWW professional wrestler The Undertaker meant that the Big Man was often photographed in India. Interesting that India is the only place where he will say yes when someone asks to take his picture.

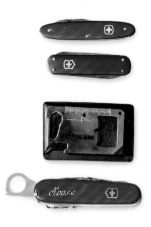

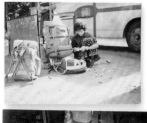

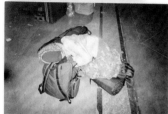

## LOT 190
### THREE SWISS ARMY KNIVES, A 'SURVIVAL AID', AND TWO PHOTOGRAPHS
$30–$40

The top photograph shows me in 1980 enjoying a roadside picnic at a bus stop in the hills of Sri Lanka. The bottom photograph shows me sleeping during a 10-hour train delay on a railway platform in Jaipur, in 2005. On both occasions, I was carrying jewellery underneath all my tatty clothing – bundles of silver-set moonstone necklaces and earrings in 1980, and various pairs of 22ct gold earrings set with diamonds and enamel in 2005, as seen in Lot 198. The green skirt is featured in Lot 101.

## LOT 191
### COLLECTION OF HANDPAINTED ENAMEL SHIVA EYES
$50–$100

Varanasi, India, 2013. Big Man and I were meandering through the ancient streets that wind up the hill from the ghats on the Ganges, when I came across the tiniest shop selling these enamel eyes. I had seen the eyes on many little orange Shivlings, aniconic forms representing creation that appear in various shapes and sizes at auspicious locations.

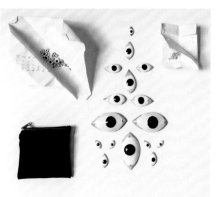

I thought these tiny eyes would be useful spares for sentimental items I regularly bought and sold, which often had eyes missing – including the 'Fums Up' dolls, mascots made to bring good luck to men fighting in World War I.

These tiny silver dolls had wooden heads (touch wood for luck) and arms articulated to give the thumbs-up signal (see Lot 195). Yet I could never bring myself to use these all-seeing eyes for such a repair, so they remain all-seeing, despite being tightly packed and muffled in their blue velvet bag.

## LOT 192
## TWO NIPPON BISQUE CHARACTER DOLLS IN ORIGINAL CLOTHES, c1920
$170–$200

These little antique child dolls are whimsical souvenirs of a trip I made to Japan with the Big Man to attend a jewellery trade show, during which time I missed my daughters.

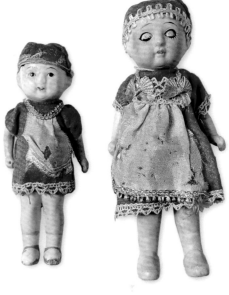

## LOT 193
## FOUR GLASS BOTTLE TOPS AND A VINTAGE FOILED GOLD-TOP MILK-BOTTLE SEAL, A DOOR KEY AND RUSTY TIN CHILD'S TOY PLATE
$5–$10

These simple items represent years of hard and rewarding work, as they are all things we have found in the Australian properties we have restored, renovated and rebuilt. The most interesting item, and also the most fragile, is a foiled gold-top seal from a glass milk bottle, which we found underneath the floorboards in my home in Newtown.

In England and Australia, through much of the 20th century, the milkman would make daily pre-dawn rounds delivering bottled milk to homes. I remember the chink-chink sound as the milk cart drove slowly along the street, as the 'empties' that had been left on the doorstep were replaced with full bottles. The concept of recycling the bottles was organic and obvious – sometimes the bottles would be really worn on the outside, yet it mattered not; it was the quality of what was on the inside that was important.

I remember the regular silver-top bottles and the more expensive, but much more delicious, gold-tops of my childhood. During winter, the milk could be left on the doorstep for some time and birds, including sparrows and robins, would poke a hole in the foil top and drink the cream that had formed on top of the milk. In the heat of summer, however, the milk would get warm and quickly turn. At primary school, we would each have to drink a small bottle of milk every morning, which was fine in winter, but in summer, both the milk, and my stomach, would churn.

Later, on Sundays at boarding school, we were treated to gold-top milk for our cornflakes. As we sat at the refectory tables in the dining room, as soon as we had finished saying grace, a cry would go up in unison from each table: "Bags the top of the milk!"

Such memories evoked by one small, inconsequential piece of rubbish.

## LOT 194
## ORANGE STONE RING SET IN SILVER, IN BOX, c1940
$20–$30

I have had this ring in my possession for an exceedingly long time. I believe it belonged to a family member, but don't recall whether she was my mother or my grandmother. It is interesting to note how this lack of personal information decreases the subjectively assumed value of an object.

For a few years in the early 2000s, I worked as a consultant to a Sydney auction house, where I was the senior specialist in the jewellery department. One of my roles was to meet with potential clients who were considering consigning jewellery for auction. Much of the jewellery had been inherited, and the estates of the deceased needed to be valued for probate purposes, or to be distributed amongst the beneficiaries. The most difficult part of my job was not calculating the value of the piece, as I had neither memories evoked by it, nor attachment to it. The difficulty was always breaking the news to the family of the estimated commercial value of these inherited treasures. My most oft-used phrase was: "It is worth more to you as a sentimental piece, a remembrance, than it is as an item to be offered for sale."

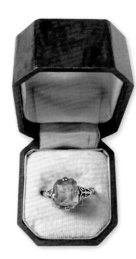

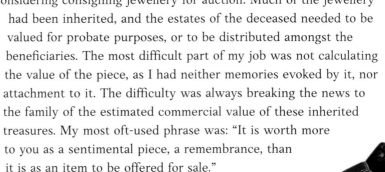

## LOT 195

### AGFACOLOR PHOTO-SLIDE BOX CONTAINING AN ASSORTMENT OF TRINKETS

$450–$500

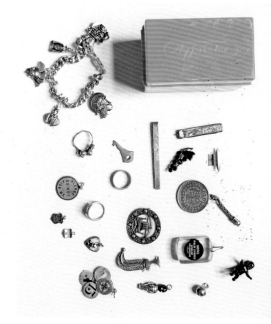

This is typical of the 'mixed lot' of items I would be asked to assess in my role as senior specialist of the jewellery department. Nothing here is of any significant value. Commercially, the most precious items are the 9ct gold Fums Up doll (bottom centre), and the early-20th-century continental silver and enamel 'Good Luck' pendant (bottom left). This, however, is my personal 'mixed lot' and herein lies the twist. All these items could be considered of 'no commercial value' (NCV), yet they have significance for me. I am torn – attachment is a curse. It is time to practise non-attachment and look within.

## LOT 196

### HANDMADE JEWELLERY ROLL AND PACKAGING, EARLY 2000s

$10–$20

The most valuable gift anyone can give me is something that's been made specifically for me. I trust I'm not alone in this self-centred appreciation. This gift is so perfect – the item, the use of recycled materials, the design, the colour, the function and presentation. So perfect a representation of love, knowledge and connection that I keep it, unused and pristine, in its original recycled wrapping.

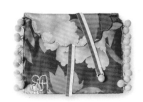

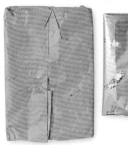

   This jewellery roll was made as a gift by Clare Bolton, a young girl with whom I was working, mentoring and sharing our daily lives whilst we ran the 'Fine' (and not so fine) jewellery department at the auction house. We came to know each other inside-out and became an incredible team, significantly raising the profile and turnover of the company, whilst quietly and powerfully watching each other's backs, taking care of one another in myriad ways.

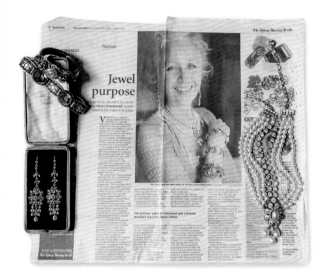

## LOT 197

**VARIOUS ITEMS OF PASTE JEWELLERY, INCLUDING A PAIR OF GEORGIAN SILVER 'HARLEQUIN' EARRINGS, IN BOX, AND NEWSPAPER CUTTING, 2004**

$1500–$2000

An article about costume jewellery featured a large photo of yours truly in *The Sydney Morning Herald*. It was a surreal experience, seeing myself in this medium.

## LOT 198

**PAIR OF 22CT GOLD EARRINGS SET WITH DIAMONDS AND TOURMALINES, WITH JAIPUR ENAMEL ON THE REVERSE, 2005, AND AN 18CT GOLD AND HINGED BANGLE SET WITH DIAMONDS, PLUS FOUR 18CT GOLD BANGLES, AND PHOTOGRAPH, c1990–2000**

$10,000–$12,000

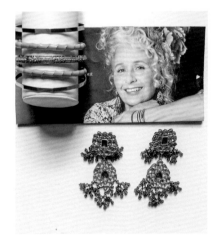

I had never heard of Botox when, later in 2004, as a result of a large photo having been in *The Sydney Morning Herald* (Lot 197, above), I was asked by a beauty company to be the face of their campaign launching this new treatment. I explained to them that my 'beauty routine' consisted merely of over-exfoliation and abundant moisturising, coupled with laughing a lot. They didn't seem to mind when I vowed there and then that I would never use this product. I had no idea of the massive impact Botox would have, not only on the beauty industry, but also people's lives and their self-esteem.

I keep my promises, and here's the shot.

These massive diamond-encrusted earrings were amongst those in my pocket whilst I was sleeping on Jaipur railway station in 2005 (see Lot 190).

## LOT 199

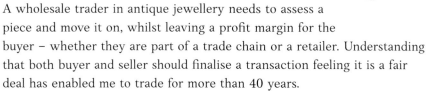

### COLLECTION OF FOUR RARE ANTIQUE SILVER LOUPES (MAGNIFYING GLASSES), 1800s–1950s, AND ONE PLASTIC TOY FROM A CHRISTMAS CRACKER (TOP CENTRE)

$1400–$1700

A wholesale trader in antique jewellery needs to assess a piece and move it on, whilst leaving a profit margin for the buyer – whether they are part of a trade chain or a retailer. Understanding that both buyer and seller should finalise a transaction feeling it is a fair deal has enabled me to trade for more than 40 years.

Knowing how many hundreds of thousands of items have passed through my hands in that time, it is incredible to consider how many important and valuable jewels have been identified and assessed using only these basic and beautiful instruments. The eye and a good loupe have always been the most important tools of the trade.

The smallest, and most recent, of these miniature magnifying glasses measures 1 inch (2.5cm) from end to end, and dates from the 1950s (centre right). The engraved piece (centre left) dates from the late 1900s, whilst the two 'scissor-mechanism' magnifiers (bottom left and right) are from the mid- to late 1800s.

The magnification of all four works well, the oldest of them being the most powerful.

## LOT 200

### TWO HANDMADE LUCKY MASCOTS: A CHAMPAGNE CORK, 1940, AND ARTICULATED BLACK CAT, c1900

$30–$50 (WITHDRAWN)

These two. Cheeky, fun, naive. No idea who made them. They came separately, but now are friends forever.

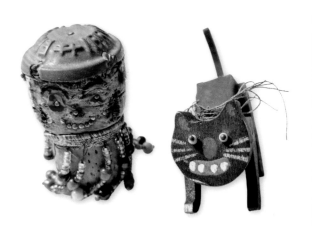

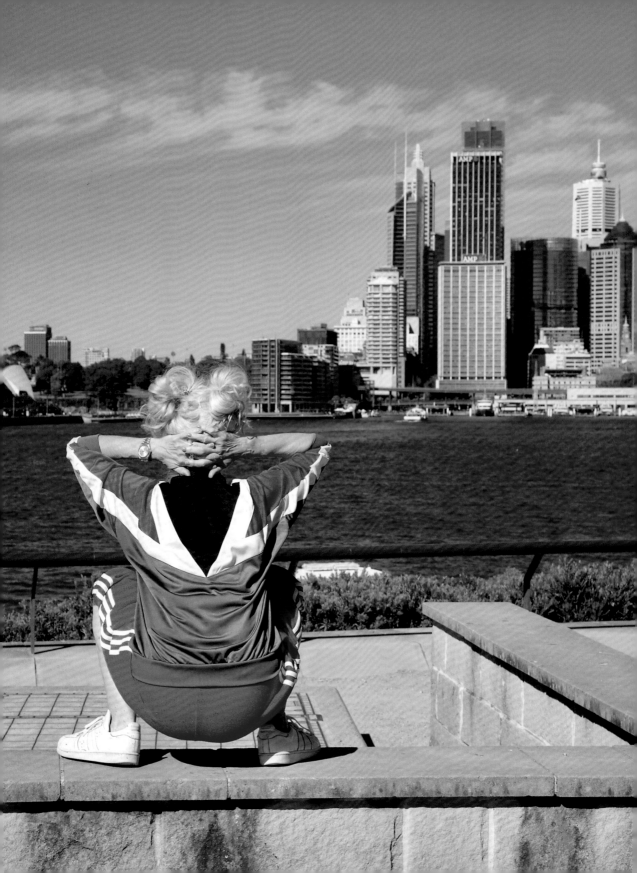

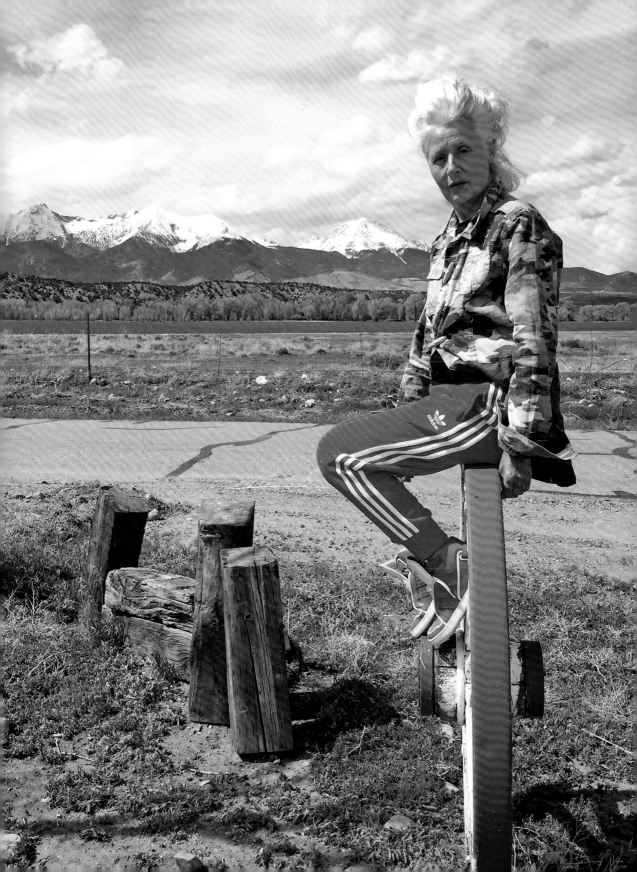

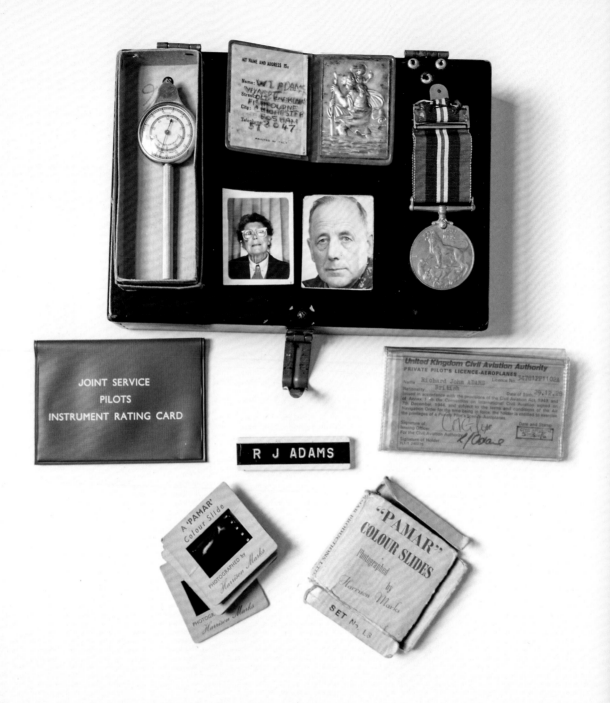

CHAPTER **13**

# change is a constant

LOT **201**

## MINIATURE SCOTCH WHISKY BOTTLE IN A MATCHBOX, 1960s, AND MINIATURE CZECH GLASS PEARS SOAP, 1920s

$100–$120

Five years into our marriage, something came over me. I was short-tempered, anxious and, for the first time in my life, teary.

Menopause.

Timing is everything – sometimes perfect, sometimes cruel. Triggers revealed a person I almost didn't recognise. A touch from the Big Man, a coffee, an annoying occurrence, a frustration – all brought on sudden, frequent, intense hot flushes. Day and night, my emotions were raw. The first two years were the worst – the Big Man and I had only been together a few years, yet I seemed to be withdrawing from him and, understandably, he felt I was losing interest.

Our conversations moved from discussing the children's wellbeing to clarifying what was happening between us. Each day, I awoke to a different understanding of who I was. Meeting and accepting this evolving person

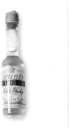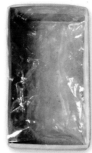 was often testing for both of us, yet, deep down, I knew that by jointly accepting this process, our commitment would transform into a different kind of partnership – long-lasting, unquestionable and true. I was daily becoming stronger, growing into the person I deserved to be. Within any relationship, this is uncharted territory. Change is a constant, and menopause is a great opportunity to press the refresh button on just about everything.

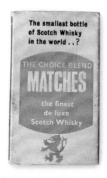

*Timing is everything – sometimes perfect, sometimes cruel.*

I chose to embrace this process naturally, as I believe menopause to be an incredibly important rite of passage that should be acknowledged and accepted as part of the transformative process in the cycle of life. My menopause has lasted a good 12 to 15 years and with love, acceptance and patience from the Big Man, I have come to understand the ever-evolving energy I am becoming. This is the time for a woman to become gracious, accepting and truly, naturally, beautiful.

These are my 'His and Hers' mementos of these times.

The matchbox containing a small novelty bottle of scotch whisky is from the 1960s Grant's Whisky Matchbox series, made by the Cumbrae Supply Company, near Glasgow. The miniature bar of Pears soap would have been a salesman's sample at a time when salesmen would travel miles to visit shops and homes, using miniatures to display their wares to their customers. Orders would be placed and deliveries sent out later. It would have been a harrowing job, described in detail in the 1949 play *Death of a Salesman*, by Arthur Miller, which was one of the works I studied for English 'A' level.

## LOT 202
## VICTORIAN GARNET BANGLE IN BOX, c1860, AND PHOTOGRAPH, 2005
$1200–$1500

The fully encrusted bangle comprises a domed central piece, flanked by wide shoulders tapering to a substantial underside, all set with rose-cut Bohemian garnets in a gold-filled setting. The more than 150-year-old bangle is seen here, worn with the 33-year-old handmade leather wrist band (Lot 63) in a photo shoot for an article in *InStyle* magazine suggesting looks for each generation. I had recently turned 50.

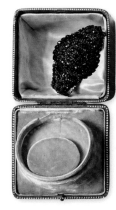

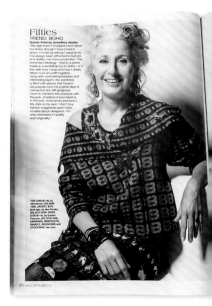

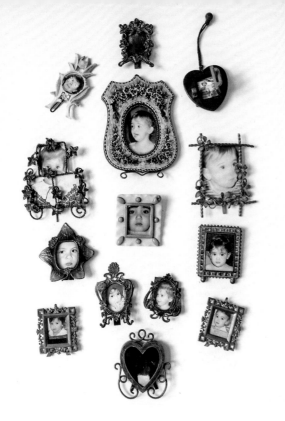

## COLLECTION OF 14 MINIATURE PHOTOGRAPH FRAMES, c1900

$1300–$1500

There are no photographs on show on the walls or shelves in my home. My stress levels rise rapidly when I enter a room with that overly cluttered look. I see only chaos and instantly feel the urge to straighten the groups of small frames holding pictures, photographs, inspirational quotes and the like, none of which I actually *see*.

So, the remedy for this is to frame my loved ones in a collection of miniature, antique and stylistically different settings. Some frames are only the size of an old postage stamp, some show art nouveau styling and some are deeply symbolic, such as the ivy ('I cling to thee'). The shape of the carved bone frame, its stand replaced by an old hair clip, resembles an edelweiss flower (see Lot 19), and it holds my beloved grandmother, Nanny Win.

LOT **204**

## PLUSHIE TOY FERRET, A BOX OF ASHES LABELLED 'BUSTER', AND OTHER EPHEMERA INCLUDING TWO PHOTOGRAPHS

$1–$5 (WITHDRAWN)

Christmas 2008 was when our family discovered our love of ferrets. To some, it was a strange choice for a family pet, but Buster the ferret lived with us for six years. This clever, stinky, loving little animal seemed to gel the family together and we became members of the ferret community.

My first foray into social media was supporting a fundraiser for those ferrets suffering from insulinoma and adrenal disease. 'Zander' was a plushie ferret that was sent to spend a week with people who donated to the cause,

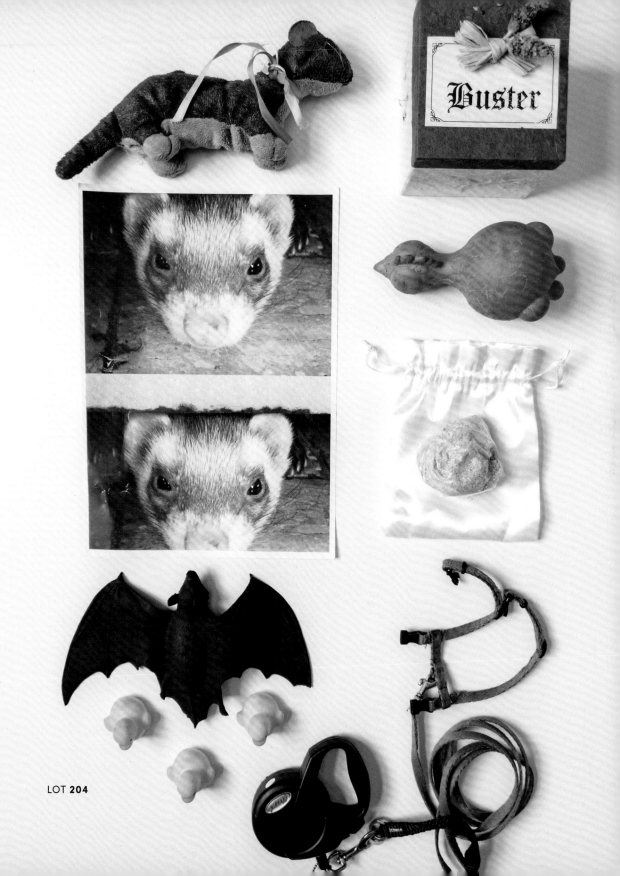

LOT **204**

their task being to document and promote Zander's time with them by posting images on social media. When we received Zander, I decided to add a little spice to his life and introduced another, smaller plushie ferret, whom we named Widdle Won (pictured on the previous page). Within a week, these two had formed an enchanting relationship, while also showcasing some of the most interesting parts of Sydney on their 'travels'. More importantly, through this process, I began to understand the power of social media and, in June 2013, when we sent Zander off to his next host family, I started an Instagram account celebrating @theadventuresofwiddlewon.

Our real ferret, Buster, was cremated in September 2014 and now rests in peace in a box alongside a few of his favourite squeaky rubber toys (pictured on the previous page). He also featured in an early post on my then newly created Instagram page, @saramaijewels, in February 2014.

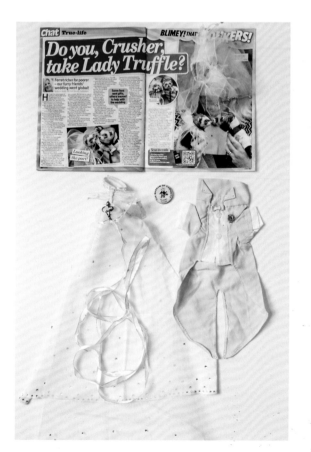

## LOT 205

### MINIATURE HANDMADE WEDDING DRESS AND GROOM'S TAIL COAT, *CHAT* MAGAZINE CLIPPING DATED 21 FEBRUARY 2013, AND BADGE, c1975

$20–$30

Our involvement in fundraising for the international ferret community brought us into contact with some real characters. One of them was a woman from the north of England, who decided to raise money by holding a 'wedding ceremony' between two of her ferrets. My contribution was a pair of 9ct gold engraved wedding bands, which I sent across to be auctioned after the event. The occasion made the tabloids and I was presented with the bride's and groom's outfits. The badge, from Potter's Museum of Curiosity, has been with me since my childhood (see Lot 38).

## LOT 206
### NIPPON BISQUE FIGURINE OF TWO KEWPIES, c1920
$250–$300

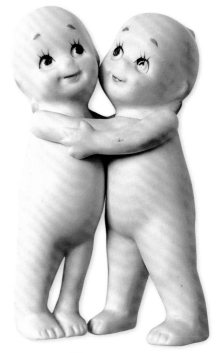

I found these twin Kewpie dolls in a flea market in Tokyo, in 2010. The name Kewpie evolved from a cupid baby who first appeared in 1909 in an illustrated cartoon strip by New Yorker Rose O'Neill. Apparently, Rose created these characters to inspire folks to be happy and kind to one another. They quickly found popularity and now Kewpie dolls are highly collectible. Of course, to me, they represent the ideal of twindom.

## LOT 207
### SPICE GIRLS DRESS, 2000s
$5–$10

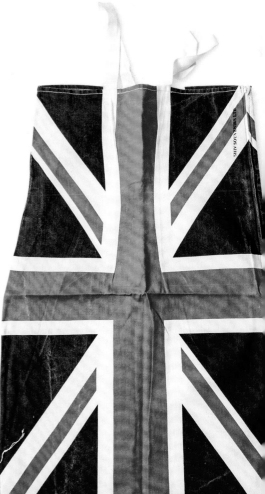

Back in the mid-1990s, the Spice Girls ruled in our household. Long after the craze had ended and my girls had moved out of home, they decided to hold a Spice Girls party. Olivia was Sporty Spice, Tash was Scary Spice... and I was invited.

Always up for a challenge and a laugh, I decided to surprise them. I bought two Union Jack tea towels and spent a couple of hours knocking up this mini dress. Wearing a cheap ginger wig, I turned up at the party – Geri had arrived. We all thought it was hilarious and – surprise, surprise – as often happens at such events, the Adams family members were the only ones who dressed up.

## LOT **208**
### FOUR BOXES CONTAINING BIRDS' EGGS, EARLY 1900s
$150–$200

Some years ago, I was wandering through an antiques centre in country Australia, when four beautiful old boxes caught my eye. Labels intact, they comprise three timber cigar boxes and a chocolate box. Drawn to these boxes, I opened the biggest to discover a collection of the most exquisite birds' eggs, nestled snugly in a soft bed of cotton wool. The name Phyllis Mary Osborn is written in childish letters in two of the boxes, and one bears the label 'Soldier Birds'. It seems that Phyllis may have been a voracious nest-robber in her day. Obviously, I do not condone such practices and never in this life would I have partaken in such behaviour. However, I wonder, had I been born in England in the late 1800s and come to Australia as a young girl, would I have also inquisitively and 'lovingly' collected these perfect forms, wrongly interpreting the act of nest-robbing as one of appreciation and learning?

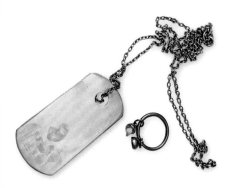

## LOT **209**
### 18CT GOLD SPLIT RING WITH TWO CHARMS (ONE TOOTH MISSING), 1999, AND 18CT GOLD 'DOG TAG' PENDANT ON CHAIN, 2005
$380–$450

These items have always been my travel companions when I am separated from my children. The charms held a milk tooth from each of my daughters, a piece of their DNA always with me. Each side of the dog tag features a laser-engraved image of my girls, aged 16.

Sentimental jewellery became popular in the 1800s. Queen Victoria wore a golden bracelet set with her children's milk teeth. She also had a gold pendant and earring suite featuring Princess Beatrice's baby teeth as the stamen of an enamel fuchsia, the flower symbolising humility and love.

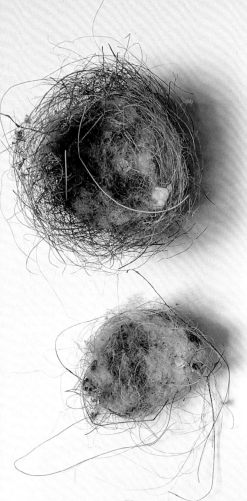

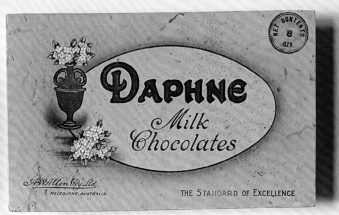

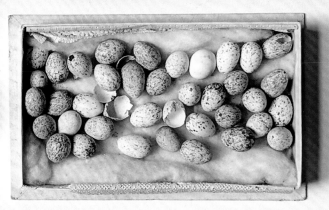

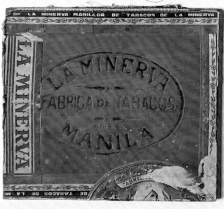

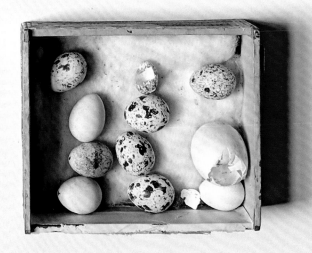

LOT **208**

LOT **210**

## COLLECTION OF JEWELLERY AUCTION CATALOGUES, 2003

$5–$10

Three years working on and off at the auction house meant that both I and the job were beginning to lose our sparkle. The jewellery department's turnover had quadrupled over that time, yet, the more we achieved, the more the bar was raised. In the throes of menopause, I did not suffer fools gladly. We were attracting more 'important' clients and one day I had to decline an unreasonable request from a particularly self-important one. When she retorted, "Why are you still working here anyway?"

I immediately felt a hot flush rise through my body, my neck and my face until I was ready to explode. Menopause had empowered me to speak my mind; instead, I held my counsel.

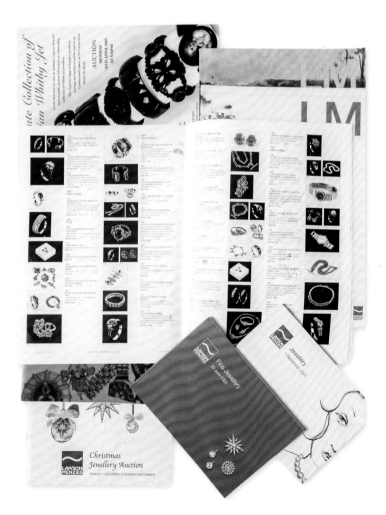

*The more we achieved, the more the bar was raised.*

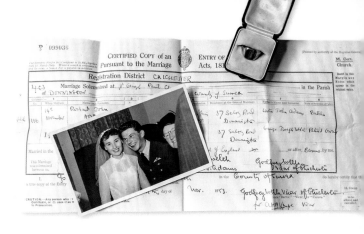

## LOT 211

**18CT GOLD GENTLEMAN'S SIGNET RING (WORN), IN BOX, PHOTOGRAPH AND CERTIFICATE OF MARRIAGE, DATED 14 NOVEMBER 1953**

$100–$150

This is my father's wedding ring. I remember his hands, oily, gnarly, always busy doing something, the ring so worn it almost became part of them. He never removed the ring, until his body became so frail and thin, and I held both those hands in mine as he took his last breaths.

## LOT 212

**HANDMADE BOX CONTAINING AN OPISOMETER IN A BOX, ST CHRISTOPHER MEDAL, SET OF PAMAR COLOUR SLIDES, ASSORTED PHOTOGRAPHS, CARD, LICENCE AND NAME TAG (SHOWN ON PAGE 230)**

$20–$40

This is my father's RAF 'Life in a Box'. I remember him planning our holiday road trips, tracing the wheel at the bottom of the opisometer across large unfurled, but still annoyingly concertinaed, maps, on the infuriatingly small kitchen table. Somehow, as that little device clicked over, he was able to work out the distances we would be driving.

I'm sure in its professional capacity, this tool helped him plan many dangerous and challenging sorties, yet I felt that my father was in his comfort zone while he used it. The restrictive size of the kitchen table clearly was not frustrating for him, compared to being mid-flight in a cramped cockpit, using a map tucked behind a perspex-covered rectangle set into the leg of his flying overalls.

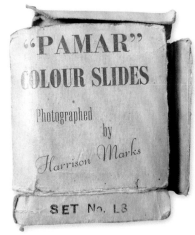

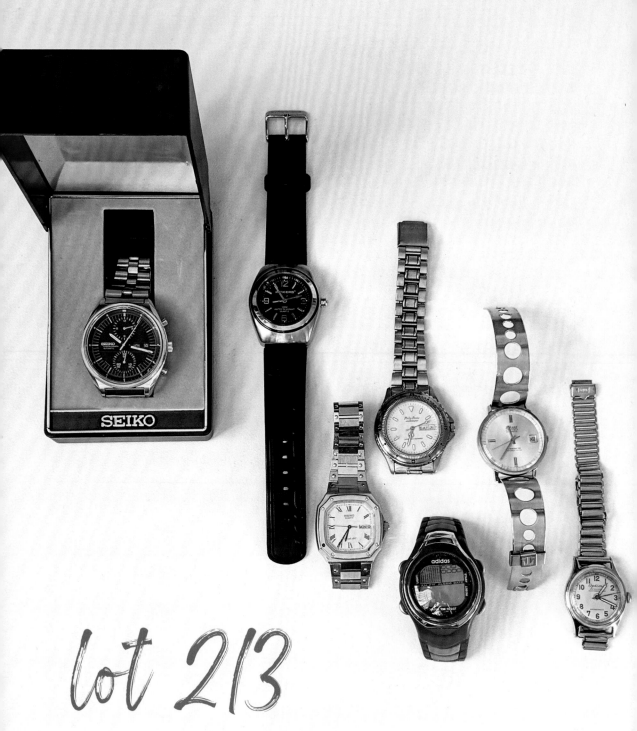

lot 213

## LOT **213**

### COLLECTION OF SEVEN WRISTWATCHES, INCLUDING A BOXED SEIKO

$300–$400

These belonged to my late father. The Optima, at bottom right, is his RAF military mechanical (hand-winding) watch, dated early 1950s. My father witnessed the transition of the wristwatch from mechanical through automatic to digital and, as an engineer and a bit of a watch freak, he was fascinated by these developments.

## LOT **214**

### BONHAMS *COLLECTORS' MOTOR CARS, MOTORCYCLES AND AUTOMOBILIA* CATALOGUE, 2005

$50–$70

My father's classic cars, which he had painstakingly restored over a number of years, found new owners, whom I feel sure would have loved them differently, through this Bonhams sale. I did not attend the sale.

I now recognise that I inherited not only my father's engineering skills, dismantling and reassembling anything and everything, but also his beady eye for detail and quality. These skills almost certainly assisted me with my early creations, and surely have been a major part of my success as an antique-jewellery dealer and jewellery designer.

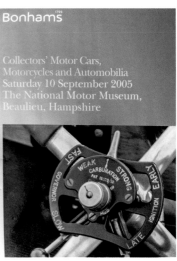

Bonhams

Collectors' Motor Cars, Motorcycles and Automobilia Saturday 10 September 2005 The National Motor Museum, Beaulieu, Hampshire

When inspecting a piece of jewellery, I mentally assess its process of manufacture, and the often-complex combinations of production methods, settings and finishes, and more. These are as important as the quality of the gemstone, its colour, cut and polish. Then there's the aesthetic, the design, the essence of a piece that cannot be described easily. Finally, what will it represent to the owner, the wearer?

So much of this is 'felt'. How do we begin to understand the different attachments people feel to objects?

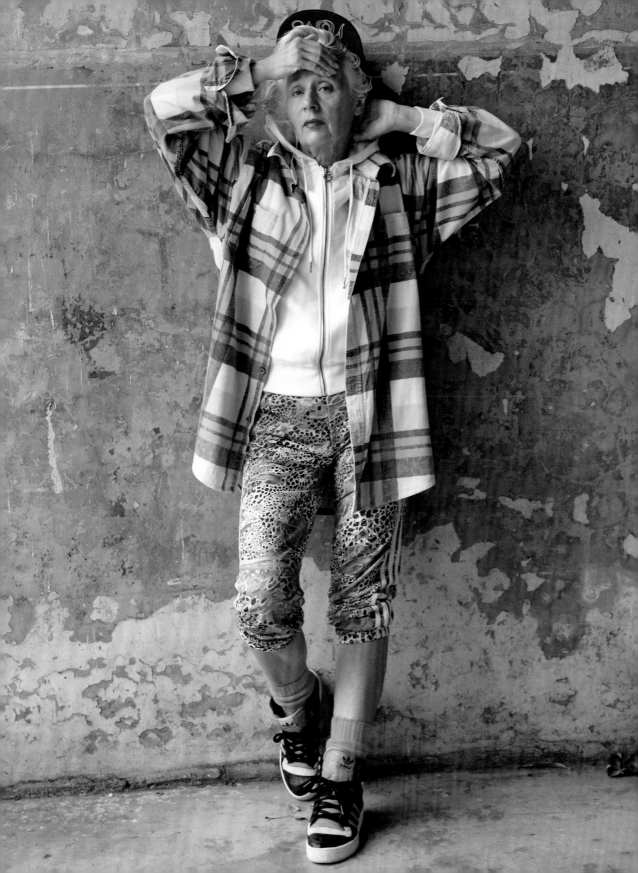

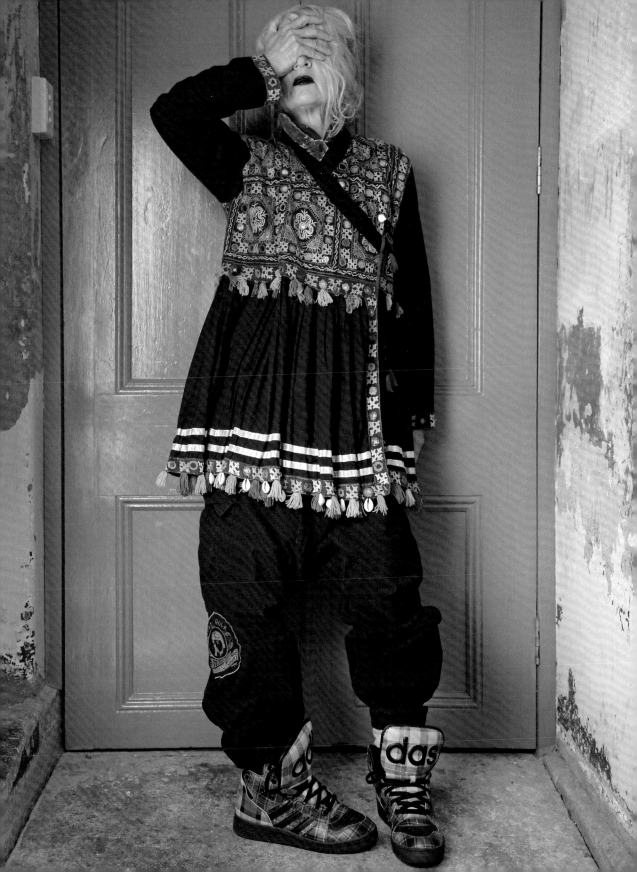

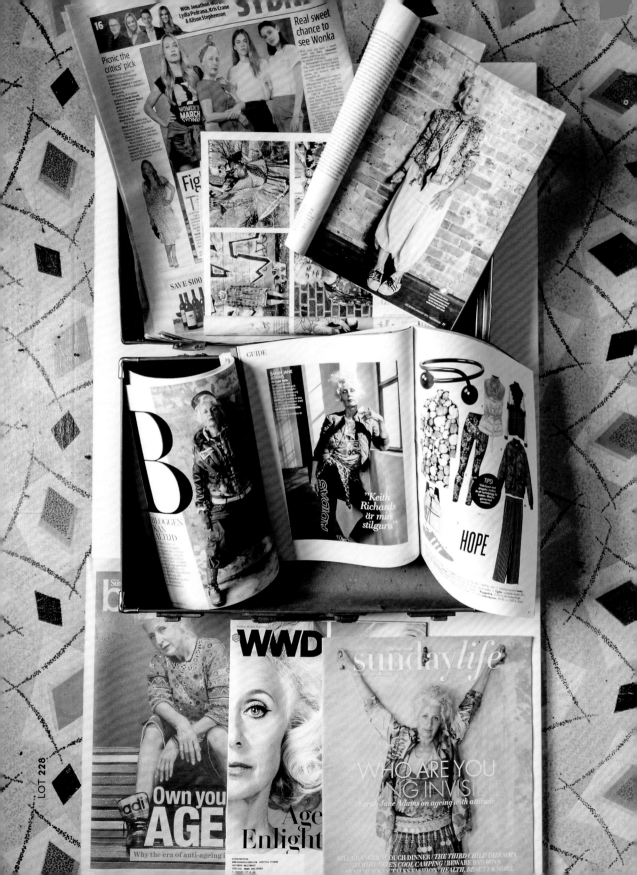

# juggling madly

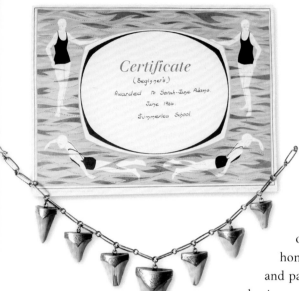

Certificate
(Beginner's)
Awarded to Sarah-June Adams
June 1964
Summerlea School

LOT **215**

## AUSTRALIAN SILVER-MOUNTED SHARK'S-TOOTH NECKLACE, c1900, AND SWIMMING CERTIFICATE, 1964

$4500–$5500

In the old days of the jewellery industry, diamonds and other precious items were held or sold on a handshake. There was integrity and honour among the trade; people kept their word and paid their bills. This was my background in the business – I borrowed nothing, paid immediately, and ran a tight ship in which my carefully selected stock stood on its own merit and needed no branding. In Australia, each of my customers was always eager to be the first to see a new collection, and it was often difficult deciding who to show first. Clients were avaricious about my stock – they knew it was all saleable, being different, beautiful, all hand-selected by me. It was always in original and perfect condition, and fully paid for.

I was also sourcing good-quality reproduction items, which were offered as such alongside my genuine antiques. Much like the game of Chinese Whispers, though, descriptions would be altered further along the chain and I became aware that some of my new items were being misrepresented as original antique pieces.

In 2005, Big Man and I launched a business, which ran parallel to my antique-jewellery business. The reasons were many: I wanted complete transparency around the origin of my newly manufactured stock; and, as tastes and demographics changed, there was now a demand for lower priced, antique-inspired jewellery. I jumped in deep, knowing I could swim among the sharks (albeit annoying them). And so, Saramai Jewels was born. I had a massive website built, saramai.com, which clearly indicated that all the items shown on it were new.

I hold my nose and always jump in at the deep end.

## 18CT GOLD HANDMADE 'CRANES' BROOCH WITH INVISIBLE-SET RUBIES, SAPPHIRES AND DIAMONDS, WHICH BREAKS INTO TWO DRESS CLIPS, 2004

$7000–$8000 (WITHDRAWN)

Saramai Jewels was born as my father was leaving us.

In the final few days of his life, this brooch came my way and my father purchased it for me. In his heavily sedated state, he spent hours and hours mesmerised by the piece, recognising not only its beauty, but, as an engineer, its spectacular craftsmanship.

The new business needed a logo, and I used this piece as the basis for the design. The sweeping curves of the birds' necks formed the 'S', the open space in the centre of the piece became the horizontal of the 'J', with the finished profile reflecting that of a round brilliant-cut diamond.

I did a few sketches, collaborated with a graffiti artist, and the SJ Jewels logo was born.

The crane is symbolic in many cultures, representing longevity and fidelity, as well as vigilance and happiness.

I revealed the story behind the inspiration for this logo in March 2014, on the business's Instagram account, @saramaijewels.

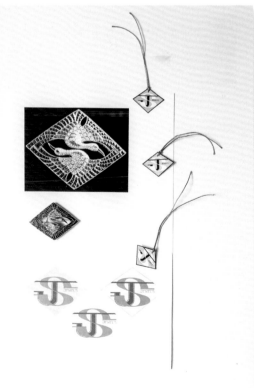

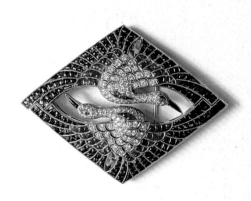

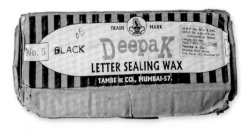

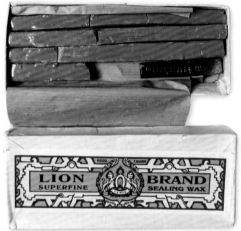

## LOT 217
### TWO BOXES OF SEALING WAX, 2004
$20–$30

For the branding of the Saramai Jewels website, I wanted to use imagery that evoked a sense of history, dependability, value and integrity, along with a sense of intimacy and secrecy. Sealing wax has been used since the Middle Ages and is still used today to verify the confidentiality and authenticity of a document. It was an obvious choice to use sealing wax combined with antique seals and signet rings in our marketing. These two boxes were bought in the business area of Fort in Mumbai.

## LOT 218
### SET OF SIX 18CT GOLD BANGLES AND TWO 'SARAMAI' SEALS, c2000
$1500–$1800

The Saramai seals were made in Mumbai. The gold bangles, with rose-gold plating, were acquired in 2000 and are yet another variation on a theme!

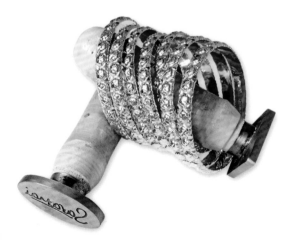

*I wanted to use imagery that evoked a sense of history, dependability, value and integrity.*

# HUMAN-HAIR GUARD CHAIN WITH 9CT GOLD FITTINGS, AND 9CT GOLD RING IN A BOX, WITH HUMAN HAIR DETAILS, c1880, AND PHOTOGRAPH, 2007

$400–$450

Before photography was commonplace, people would keep a lock of hair as a memento of a loved one. In Victorian times women would weave hair, often from a 'dearly departed', into jewellery, which is now known as 'mourning jewellery'. The guard chain is a fine example of this. The ring has the inscription 'In memory of SJ' engraved into the shield atop the band of hair.

In 2007, whilst in Turkey on a trip seeking artisans with whom to work, we visited this remarkable cave in Cappadocia, which holds a collection of more than 1600 cuttings of women's hair.

In the mid-1970s, a local potter, Chez Galip, when farewelling a female friend, asked her to leave him something to remember her by. The woman cut off a lock of her hair and gave it to him. Chez hung it in his pottery shop in Avanos and, from then on, women who visited the shop would leave him a lock of theirs, together with a note. His collection grew to such a size that, in 1979, he opened a museum at the back of his pottery shop.

I also left a lock of my hair with a note. As I was leaving the cave, I looked back to see the local guide who had taken me there, and who I could tell had taken a shine to me, surreptitiously, and with a wink, writing something on the back of my note.

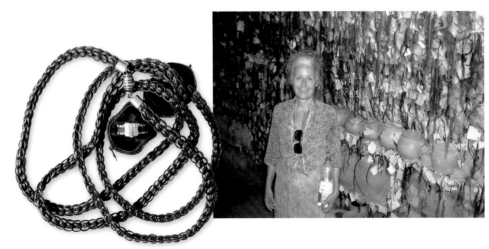

## BAG OF SJ JEWELS TIE-ON PRICE TAGS

NCV (WITHDRAWN)

I had always been fiercely against advertising, and still firmly believe that items should sell on their merit rather than marketing. So, when my daughters told me about a new platform, Instagram – one over which I would have complete creative control – I agreed to give it a go. The first @saramaijewels post went live on 11 November 2013, with the brand tagline #WhispersofthepastAspirationsoftoday.

LOT **221**

## 12 ASSORTED VESTA CASES, c1880–1905

$1500–$2000 (WITHDRAWN)

In the early days of my business, my father would sometimes accompany me to antiques fairs, where he would mooch around, looking at everything on display. Attracted to small, interesting and well-made items, it was soon decided that he would collect Vesta cases. In the 1900s, smoking was highly fashionable and popular, and, before the days of cigarette lighters, these boxes were made to hold and protect the highly flammable matches. The cases came in a variety of shapes, metals, designs and quality – from superb 18ct gold, gem-encrusted examples, to the lowly base-metal advertising variety.

My father's collection consisted of hundreds of incredible specimens. Every quality, genre, material and influence was covered in this miniature portable history lesson. I continue to buy fine examples when they cross my path. Those photographed here are as follows:

- Hallmarked sterling silver (HMSS) enamel race horse, Birmingham, 1899
- HMSS and enamel Shakespeare, Birmingham, 1908
- HMSS A Match for You, c1900 (marks worn)
- HMSS and enamel ballerina, c1900 (marks worn)
- HMSS Royal Exchange Assurance, Birmingham, 1909
- HMSS snooker, Birmingham, 1884
- HMSS bulldog, Birmingham, 1909
- HMSS golfing, Chester, 1903
- Plus, four Victorian brass cases: a glove, Huntley & Palmers biscuit, sailor and lifebuoy, and man sitting in an outdoor 'dunny'.

# Lot 220

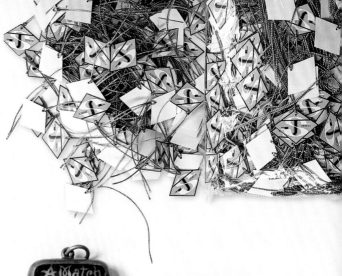

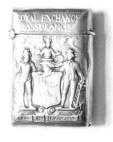
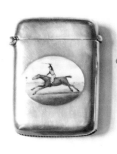
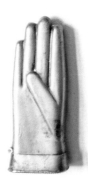
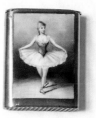
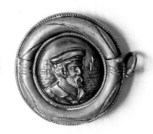
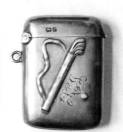
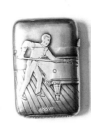
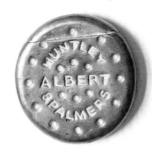
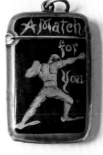
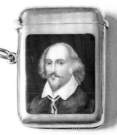
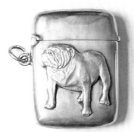
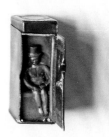

LOT **221**

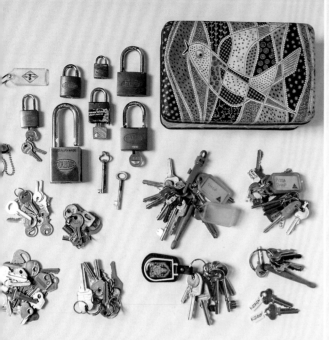

LOT **222**

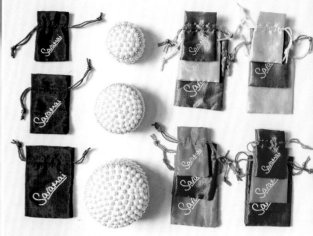

LOT **223**

LOT **224**

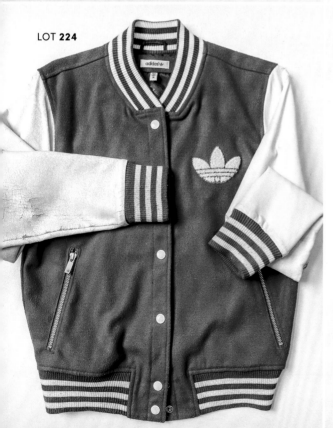

LOT **225**

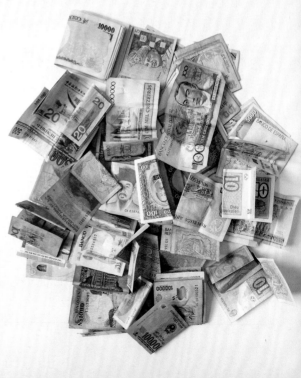

LOT **222**

## VINTAGE TIN, c1950, CONTAINING ASSORTED KEYS AND PADLOCKS

$20–$40

This tin holds keys to some of the roles that, for many years I was juggling madly – property owner, traveller, jewellery designer, supplier and safe keeper. The years rolled by – ridiculously long, stressful days, with Big Man and I frequently working together into the night as we lost track of time, swept along on the crest of the booming business. We became aware that with success – and the responsibilities, pressures and expectations it entailed – we were drowning and gradually losing track of ourselves. We began to question why we were doing this.

LOT **223**

## BOXES AND POUCHES FOR SARAMAI JEWELLERY

NCV (WITHDRAWN)

Our second Instagram post, dated 9 December 2013, shows these bags with the simple statement: *"Saramai pouches all come with treasures!"*

LOT **224**

## ADIDAS COLLEGIATE-INSPIRED JACKET, SIZE 14

$30–$40

This red wool and polyester jacket with vinyl sleeves was a gift from my daughter, Olivia, in 2013. She purchased it from JD Sports in England.

LOT **225**

## BOX OF BANK NOTES FROM VARIOUS COUNTRIES, 1970s–2000s

$250–$350

A collection of leftover cash from all the places I've visited, saved in the hope of returning one day...

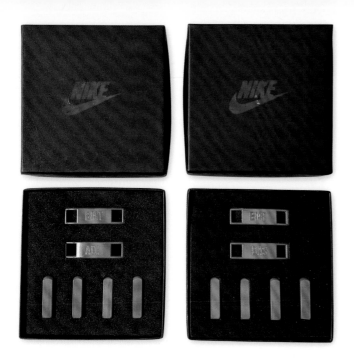

LOT 226

## TWO NIKE BOXES OF PERSONALISED SHOELACE CHARMS ENSCRIBED WITH ADI-DAS BMT-BMT

$30 - $50

Once upon a time I attended a Nike function where they were making customised shoelace charms. We were restricted to one pair per person, and I hatched a plan. Big Man is now known as BMT. Easy. I wasn't interested in SJA, as I have waaaaay too many things with my name or initials on them already. I'll never wear these babies. Wonder which team would appreciate the irony the most?

LOT 227

## SELECTION OF AMERICANA, INCLUDING VINTAGE BASEBALL SHIN GUARDS, c1950–2015

$60–$70

My obligatory souvenirs from America.

On 25 April 2015, I made my first trip to the USA, where I reconnected with Ari Seth Cohen and a friendship was forged. I have visited a number of times since.

In the late 1950s, television had been my peek into another world. The world of 'cowboys and Indians' was by far the most tantalising, as there were real people rather than puppets on the screen. Although I had not a clue what the stories were about (I still can't follow even a slightly complicated feature film), the characters in *The Lone Ranger*,

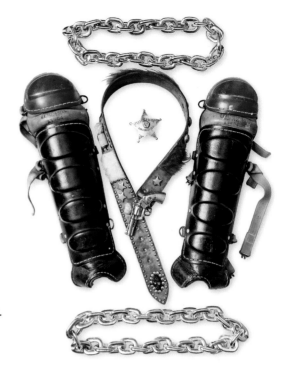

*Wagon Train* and *Tales of Wells Fargo* became my heroes. For months on end, I would only dress in my cowboy outfit and only answer to the name Jim, after Jim Hardie from the latter. My mother tells a story of how one night she woke to the sound of someone rummaging through the kitchen drawers. As she crept down in the darkness (my father was probably away night-flying), she was terrified by a voice saying, "Stick 'em up!"

It was me, the cowboy, aged about five, with both 'guns' drawn.

The chains pictured came from Las Vegas; the shin guards from a flea market in New York.

## LOT **228**
## SELECTION OF MAGAZINES AND PRESS CUTTINGS, 2015–2019 (SHOWN ON PAGE 246)
$1–$5

As I noted earlier (see Lot 140), I haven't purchased a magazine or newspaper since the 1980s. The ones pictured are the exception to my rule, as I'm in them or on the cover.

## LOT **229**
## FIVE PAIRS OF SILVER EARRINGS
$500–$800

The Big Man and I were in it together. One without the other, the business would have failed, but as a team we were indomitable. I was front-of-house, the eyes and jewellery knowledge, while he photographed all the stock and worked on the inventory. For several years, we travelled the world searching for jewellers and artisans to work with, and drove the length and breadth of Australia finding new retailers for this new version of a jewellery business.

Our customers were a different breed from the antiques dealers. Many were shopkeepers who had lucked out by jumping onto the personalised

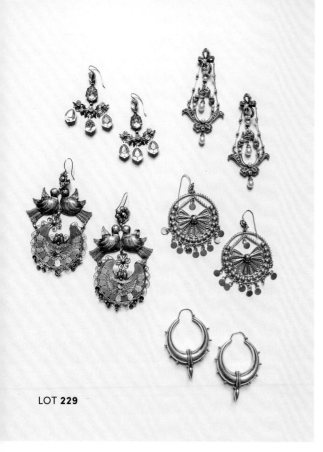

LOT **229**

jewellery trend. They had no prior knowledge where the designs in the Saramai collections had come from, pricing solely on a formula rather than understanding and appreciating the integrity of a piece. Frequently, they were more interested in the 'in-store display' and packaging than the items they were selling! I often felt I may as well have been selling sausages. The business grew and grew and grew.

I knowingly self-sabotage every few years. One day, I had simply had enough. It was time – my way of keeping things fresh. I took stock of our lives, our situation and the ridiculous hours we were working, and walked away from the business. Only one pair of these earrings became part of my stock collection; the others are trinkets bought on our travels.

LOT **230**

## COLLECTION OF 22CT GOLD BANGLES

$16,500–$18,000

I have collected these bangles, my final, grown-up set, on various trips to India, where, in Mumbai, I am always thrilled to visit the Zaveri Bazaar, marvelling at the 22ct gold jewellery, whilst searching out tools, knowledge and inspiration. The scarf was my grandmother's (see Lot 178).

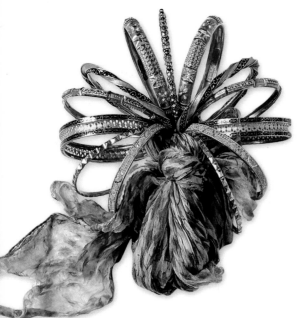

## LOT 231

## GREEN PASTE SILVER-SET BRACELET, AND HANDMADE CUFF BANGLE USING RECYCLED MATERIALS

$80–$100 (WITHDRAWN)

When someone gives a gift that once belonged to their dearest loved one, it is beyond words. The green paste bracelet is one such gift.

Ari Seth Cohen is the creator of the Advanced Style blog. He is the major instigator of the massive shift in attitudes towards ageing that we have seen in the past 10 years. Ari gave me this sweet, bright-green treasure in 2015, the day after I arrived in NYC for the first time. The bracelet had once belonged to Ari's beloved grandmother, Grandma Bluma.

In New York, Ari introduced me to Debra Rapoport, an incredible artist who was holding a workshop crafting jewellery from recycled materials. Engrossed in making this cuff, I was transported back to the simple beginnings of my life in the jewellery business. In some sense, life is coming full circle, akin to having created a major knitted piece, which now I am in the process of unpicking, unravelling and quietly, methodically, rolling back into a ball. It's simply a process. With a few interruptions along the way.

## LOT 232

## ALABASTER MODEL OF THE TAJ MAHAL, IN PRESENTATION BOX, 2015, AND AUCTION DETAILS FOR A HOUSE AND CONTENTS SALE, 2015

$50–$100

I sold my very own painstakingly restored and furnished Taj Mahal in 2015. The children had moved out and Big Man and I had, for many years, been working ridiculously long hours with Saramai Jewels. I was over it. As in, over *everything* – my customers, the huge house, the Newtown neighbourhood where I had lived for 30 years and which had changed so dramatically. Although hugely 'successful', I took stock of my life and realised it was time for a massive shift. I wanted out.

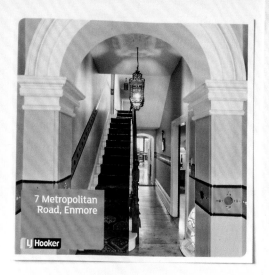

7 Metropolitan Road, Enmore

LJ Hooker

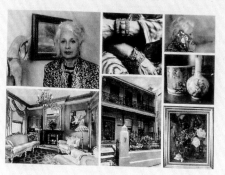
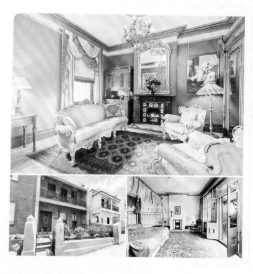

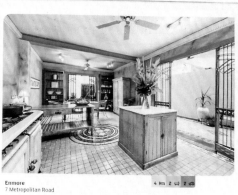

Enmore
7 Metropolitan Road

Magnificent Victorian Residence, Fine Family Living

Enjoying a quiet yet central location 'Namma' is a grand freestanding Victorian residence, one of a rare few to provide expansive living for the entertaining family.

Exquisitely restored throughout, its stunning original features have been brought back to their former glory whilst individual style has resulted in a home with a rich personality. Enjoying a choice of elegant living spaces and a superb European inspired sun trap courtyard it is further complimented by its exceptional setting an easy strol to a vast array of amenities.

Auction Sat 28th Feb 2015 at 10:00am On Site
View As advertised on our website
ljhooker.com.au/newtown
Contact: Aisling Brady 0404 066 200

LJ Hooker Newtown 9595 1888

ljhooker.com.au

Residential | Commercial | Rural | Finance

LOT **232**

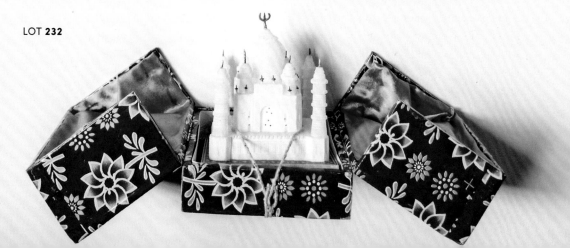

Everyone thought I had completely lost the plot, but, in fact, I was experiencing a great sense of freedom and empowerment, having almost finished a natural menopause. I knew it was time to get rid of many of my possessions and prepare for the next phase of life.

I had, both personally and at auction, witnessed so much torment and pain suffered by people who had inherited and had to sort out 'dead people's stuff'. I saw being left with the process of having to clear a deceased estate as an act of violence and as I was now entering the 'third trimester' of my life, I absolutely did not wish to inflict that on my children. By the end of March, the house and most of the contents had been sold at auction. The liberation I experienced was indescribable.

## LOT 233
## TRADITIONAL BALOCHI DRESS, WITH HANDWRITTEN NOTE AND RING (AS FOUND), c1980s
$20–$30

In February 2016, I bought this second-hand balochi dress from an Afghani nomadic trader. I found the little note and small ring in the depths of the pocket, carefully wrapped in the remnants of a plastic bag. The connection with the previous wearer of this garment is amplified by this find. Not only did the dress hold her DNA, her shape, her story, but I had a clearer memento to research.

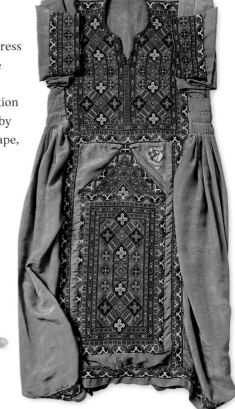

The note translates roughly as: "I wish for my children and family to stay together after me."

This is one reason I choose to wear the authentic rather than the pastiche. The connection is strong and vital. I truly believe this little amulet was sent to me for a reason.

I hope the previous owner will see this and know that my thoughts are with her. I would love her to contact me – we have so much to share.

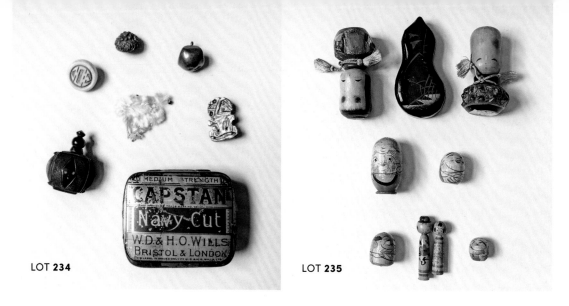

LOT **234**

LOT **235**

## LOT **234**

### CAPSTAN NAVY CUT TOBACCO TIN, c1900, CONTAINING MISCELLANEOUS ITEMS, INCLUDING A CARVED SCENT BOTTLE AND BUTTONS, c1920

$80–$100

The treasure here is the flattened, bedraggled yellow chenille blob, rediscovered squashed between two sheets of linoleum during a major renovation in 2018 of my grandparents' former home in Chichester. In my mind's eye, I still see a fluffy baby chick with her two black beady eyes and pink legs intact. I see her in her prime and my heart flutters as I recall the excitement of receiving her atop an Easter egg more than 50 years ago. The vintage buttons include Chinese and Indian silver, and a paua shell Tiki from New Zealand.

## LOT **235**

### COLLECTION OF JAPANESE MINIATURE WOODEN ITEMS INCLUDING KOKESHI DOLLS AND STACKING DOLLS, AND LACQUER BOX, c1920

$180–$250

These tiny wooden kokeshi and stacking dolls were the inspiration for a jewellery collection I designed, The Confidante Dolls (see Lot 236).

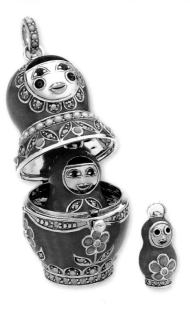

## LOT **236**
## THE CONFIDANTE DOLLS, HANDSET 925-GRADE SILVER, ENAMEL AND ASSORTED GEMSTONES
VARIOUS PRICES, COMPLETE SET $750

This is a collection I designed some years ago, which has been in hibernation. The craziness of the past few years has meant I have not been able to give it the attention it deserves.

### About the Confidante Dolls

You have a secret. Who can you trust it with? Your Confidante Doll!

She is the keeper, the protector. She passes her gift to the child – every child.

She teaches us to trust, to believe, to confide, to share. The world of woman. Confidante and protector. The keeper of the secret.

The Confidante Dolls can be interchanged, layered or worn separately. Each Mother and Daughter Doll may be used as a locket to hold your secret.

Presently there are three models of Confidante Doll.

Each set of Dolls comprises a Mother Doll, Daughter Doll and Baby Doll.

The Baby sits snugly inside the Daughter or may be worn separately as a pendant or charm. The Daughter, in turn, fits inside the Mother. She also may be worn separately.

The Mother sits snugly in the palm of the hand. She holds, and is, your secret.

The Dolls are made in 925-grade silver, and feature enamel of various colours and finishes. They are handset with freshwater pearls, natural gemstones and marcasites. Their eyes are either emerald or sapphire, and their costumes are decorated with pearls, blue topaz, turquoise...

### History of the Dolls

These pendants not only evoke the Russian matryoshka stacking dolls, but also Japanese kokeshi dolls. Kokeshi-making is a Japanese folk-art tradition dating back to the 1600s. It is believed that originally, they were a gift to ensure a healthy child, although they were also used as charms to prevent fire and ward off evil. Today, they are given as tokens of love and friendship.

Interestingly, the kokeshi was thought to have been the original inspiration for the Russian matryoshka, which was first carved in 1890. Although initially the Russian nesting doll depicted a mother and children, today, they are also made to represent contemporary culture in myriad ways. The dolls display a harmony of tradition given a modern interpretation; a treasure perfect for women in today's world.

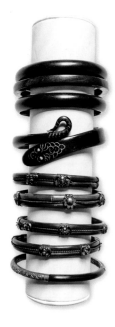

## LOT 237
## FIVE ANTIQUE CHINESE RATTAN AND SILVER BANGLES, c1900, AND FOUR VARIOUS BROWN BANGLES
$650–$750

My grandmother believed in the power of a copper bracelet to stave off her rheumatism. Traditional folklore has it that the Chinese have worn bamboo and silver bangles such as these for the same purpose. If I ever suffer from rheumatism, these will be my first remedies.

In the meantime, I adore the combination of the flexible bamboo, bent into a circle and decorated with symbolic silver bats to represent the Chinese five blessings; long life, love of virtue, good health, wealth, and finally, a peaceful death. Wonderful wishes represented in an antique circular bangle with no ending and no beginning.

## LOT 238
## PERSONALISED NECKLACE WITH ASSORTED VINTAGE SILVER AND 9CT GOLD CHARMS ON VARIOUS LENGTHS OF SILVER AND GOLD CHAIN
$1000–$1200

My idea of personalised jewellery looks like this – gold and silver charms, grouped on a tangle of chains to be worn in a variety of ways. Each item represents an aspect of my life:

- The enamel English rose charm, scissors and kangaroo signify cutting ties with England as I move to Australia.
- My children are represented here by their milk teeth, a violin, a drum and a snail.
- The tiny heart, music staff and radio: music.

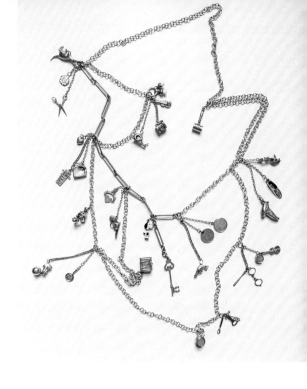

- The football, bottle openers, handcuffs and baton: Big Man.
- The safe, key, magnifying glass and auction gavel: jewellery work and business.
- Two round discs – one engraved with the 'Lord's Prayer', one with an excerpt from the Koran – suspended on a sliding silver chain: the world.
- The snake charmer: India.

LOT **239**

### *HEAT AND DUST*, BY RUTH PRAWER JHABVALA, FIRST PUBLISHED IN 1975, 'SARAMAI' 18CT GOLD RING, AND GERMAN FIGURINE OF SHIVA, c1900

$1200–$1500

Last writes. A question of identity.

In 1983, I watched the film *Heat and Dust*, set in India during the 1920s. The book, and subsequent film, tell the story of Olivia (played by Greta Scacchi), a young Englishwoman married to a British Civil Servant, who is based in Colonial India. Olivia becomes entranced not only by the country, but also by the people (the Nawab in particular), until eventually, Olivia becomes a recluse living in the foothills of the majestic Himalayan mountains.

Suffice it to say, this was a major influence on my life choices both at that time, subsequently, and in the present.

Now, like the older Olivia, I am preparing to 'head for the hills'.

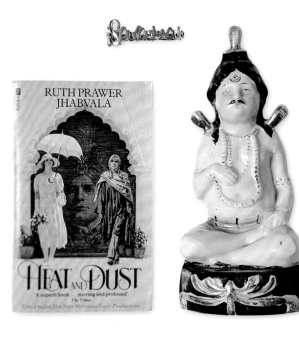

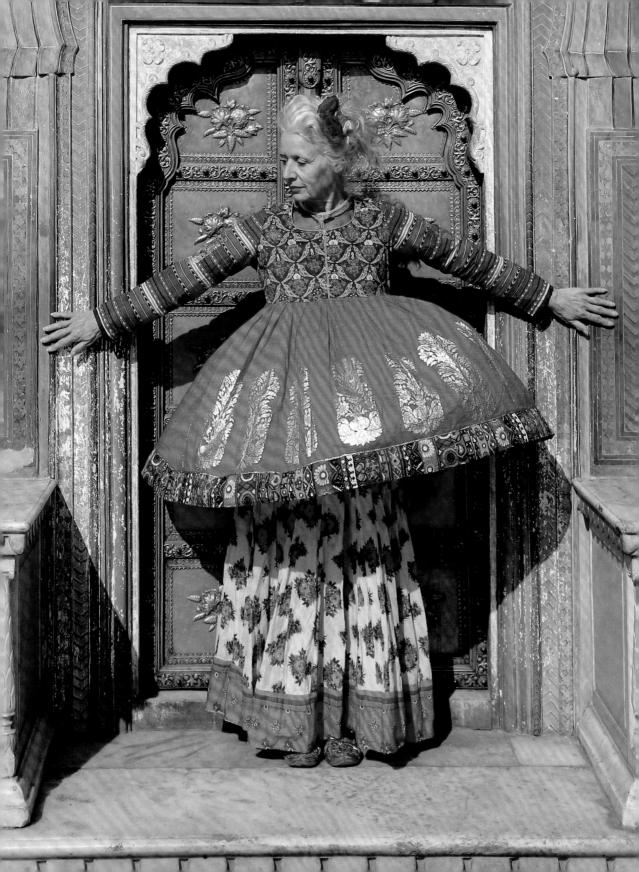

# my wrinkles are my stripes

## LOT **240**

## THE SUTHERLAND DIAMOND AWARD (BOXED SILVER MEDALLION), 2000, AND TWO FACE-CREAM SAMPLES

$30–$50

In 2000, I completed my FGAA gemmological studies by undertaking a Diploma of Diamond Technology and was awarded this medal for gaining a distinction with the highest marks.

In December 2014, I created the hashtag #mywrinklesaremystripes.

I subsequently penned this piece for *Advanced Style: Older and Wiser*, published in 2016 as a follow-up book to *Advanced Style*, also produced by Ari Seth Cohen:

*"My Wrinkles Are My Stripes*

*I love diamonds. Not so much because they sparkle and scintillate, but also for their astounding physical properties, which have a gazillion uses. So, yesterday in Sydney when I was offered a little diamond-shaped sachet on the street, how could I say no! Before I could say, 'Make mine a 3CT D VVS,' I was whisked into a store, where a delightful young lady approached me and put a blob of something onto the back of her hand.*

*'I'm just going to apply this to your eyes,' she says.*

*'Um, but what will it do?' I ask.*

*'It will completely remove all your wrinkles for approximately one week,' I'm told.*

*At this point I grab my bag, and politely tell her that actually I love my wrinkles and have no desire to get rid of them. Thank you. Maybe diamonds aren't a girl's best friend after all."*

It was on that day that I decided I had to put my hashtag #mywrinklesaremystripes out there.

The hashtag started as a tongue-in-cheek reference to the fact that I am considered by many to be too old to dress in some of my favourite clothes. As you may know, almost every day I proudly wear my three Adidas stripes. In the military, the higher the rank, the more stripes are worn.

I regularly post pictures of myself that are bare-faced, untouched and truly show my face. My clothes reveal what is going on in my head. My wrinkles do not scare me; they show me and therefore my experience.

Hopefully, there is a little wisdom that comes with these stripes. I see them as a badge of honour – as marks of roads travelled and experiences had. Why would I not be proud and happy to show them?

I am growing into the face I deserve, the face that reflects who I am and what I have been. It is not a mask. I am not a puppet.

I have been overwhelmed by the response to these posts – particularly the response from young women. I never thought of myself as inspirational; rather, the renegade. It seems, however, that there is a new generation of folks out there who are learning to accept themselves for who and what they are. This exhilarates me and drives me on with my mission.

Accept your true self, love your true self, smile and laugh often, and gather those laughter lines and creases that come when you share a joke. They are you. The world needs to see more of *you*.

## ORIGINAL PHOTO, RE-SHOT FOR ADVANCED STYLE INSTAGRAM POST, AUGUST 2014 (SHOWN OVERLEAF)

In August 2014, nine months after I had launched the Saramai Jewels Instagram account, I posted the first photo of myself (taken by the Big Man) wearing my favourite red Adidas jacket, with the words: *"So far today I've been told I look like someone from #Grease and #Dorothy from #thewizardofoz. And it's only 10.00."*

My daughter, Tash, reposted it, using the hashtags #mymumiscoolerthanme and #AdvancedStyle. I was bemused when, later that day, I received an email from Ari Seth Cohen, the New York-based founder of the Advanced Style blog, asking if he could re-shoot the photograph. I had never heard of Advanced Style, but, coincidentally, Ari was in Sydney promoting his soon-to-be-released documentary of the same name. The following day, Ari posted his own version of this photograph on Instagram, and later, on his return to New York, he wrote a little of our meeting on his blog.

In early October, the image was reposted with my permission by Adidas Originals, and I watched the 'likes' grow exponentially as the world awoke. For reasons I still don't quite understand, it went viral.

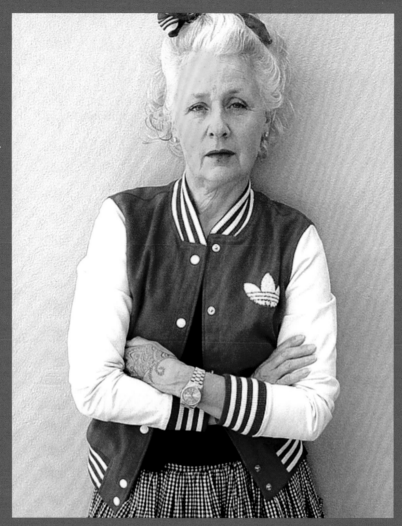

So far today I've been told I look like someone from #Grease and #Dorothy from #thewizardofoz. And it's only 10.00.

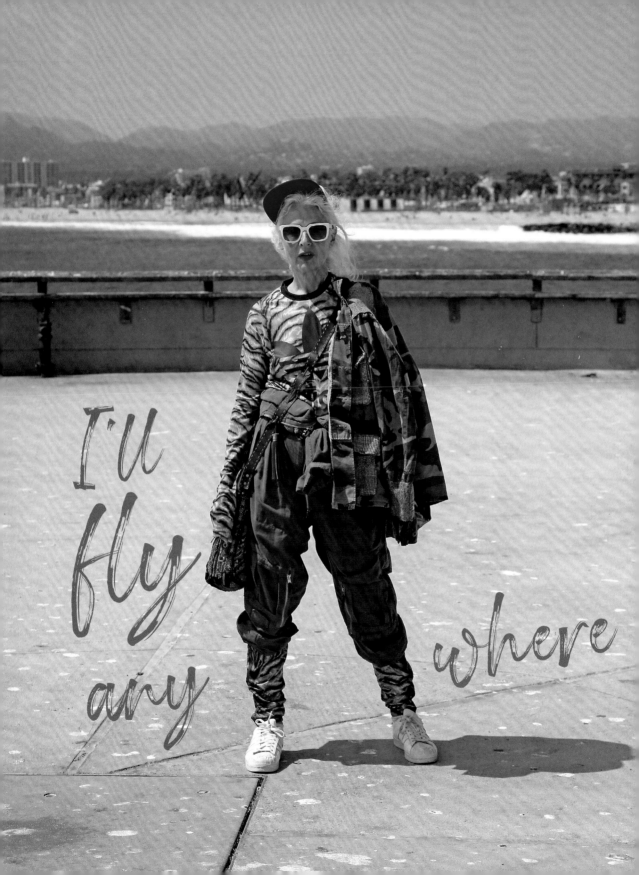

## I'LL FLY ANYWHERE, INSTAGRAM POST, MAY 2016, PICTURED IN MY FATHER'S RAF OVERALLS, VENICE BEACH, CALIFORNIA

Through my Instagram profile and online in newspapers and blogs, people were asking me about my clothing. How strange, I thought.

Here are some other thoughts:

My body shape – along with my lifestyle and attitude, and a childhood spent in school uniform – means that I never, ever, wear tailored clothing.

Our clothing is, indeed, a second skin. Mine has served as my home, my protector, my form of self-expression, my camouflage and my messenger. Within any context, I remain ambiguous, often using cross-cultural and/or cross-gender references, transitioning between gender and identity. Specific looks, but with my own clarity, the connotation of which has, more often than not, been unclear to others. Indeed, at times, I have knowingly directed misleading, or incorrect assumptions about myself through my clothing. On first impression people may find me confusing.

I have used this technique in my business, as the reality behind the apparently chaotic, hot mess is a determined and serious businesswoman.

## VITRUVIAN WOMAN, INSTAGRAM POST, JUNE 2016

This image has become a meme for numerous 'inspirational' quotes. I posted it with the words: *"Filling the Frame. Vitruvian Woman."*

My response to the person who turned me into a meme: #whodunnit

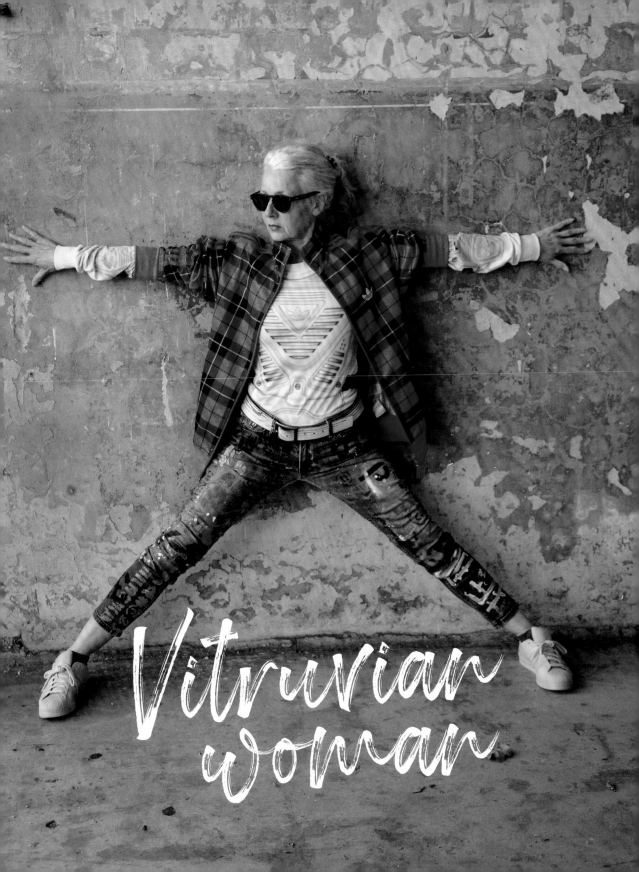

Vitruvian woman

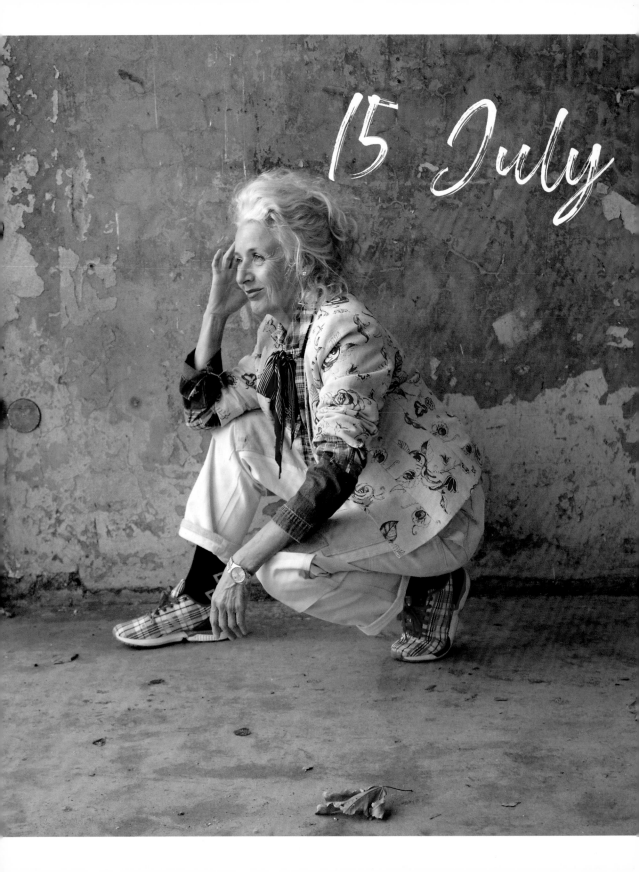

15 July

## A FEW THINGS I NEED TO SAY TODAY,
## INSTAGRAM POST, SYDNEY, JULY 2016

*"There's a few things I need to say today.*

*This 'public journey' of mine started around 18 months ago, when my first ever personal photo was spotted and re-shot by Advanced Style. Very quickly, things gathered momentum; fast forward to yesterday, when I was featured by Instagram.*

*I want to thank my husband, who takes most of my pics, my children, who, like me, have been bemused by the reactions, my friends, followers, admirers, critics, haters, basically everyone who has been with me, and against me, on this crazy ride. I represent only myself.*

*What started as an interesting way to talk about my jewellery influences, soon became a social experiment, then a form of therapy, a daily diary, a creative outlet, and a series of visuals with my thoughts and opinions.*

*I have met some incredible people and had some amazing experiences along the way. Thank you to all who have crossed my path and enriched my life.*

*Have a wonderful day. And a big welcome to all my new followers.*
*Sarah xx"*

## WORKING IT LIKE A BOSS, INSTAGRAM POST, AUGUST 2016

It seemed weird to me, this public obsession with what I wear. Here is a rare response.

*"You aren't expected to read all this, but for those of you who ask the questions, just this once, here's a detailed answer.*

*Winter has arrived and it's cold, potentially with rains coming later. (Under the shirt I'm wearing an old cotton T-shirt, and under the trousers I am wearing Adidas tracksuit pants, both for warmth.)*

*The jacket and big boots protect me from the wet and are easy to move in. I am running around doing business errands all day and need to be comfortable and armed-up against the elements and for some of the tasks in store.*

*Working it like a BOSS.*

*This is a protective, strong look, reflecting my attitude for the day. Don't mess.*

*Snapback purchased in Coney Island NYC, cost approx $30*

*Jacket purchased from Sydney flea market 10 years ago, cost approx $100*

*Shirt purchased from @raoof.atelier, cost $30*

*Tattered T shirt of my father's from the Riley Club Centenary 1998, cost £10*

*Adidas track pants from Sydney Adidas Originals, cost $75*

*Turkish trousers purchased in Istanbul 8 years ago, cost approx $35*

*New Rock boots purchased in London mid-1990s, cost approx £75"*

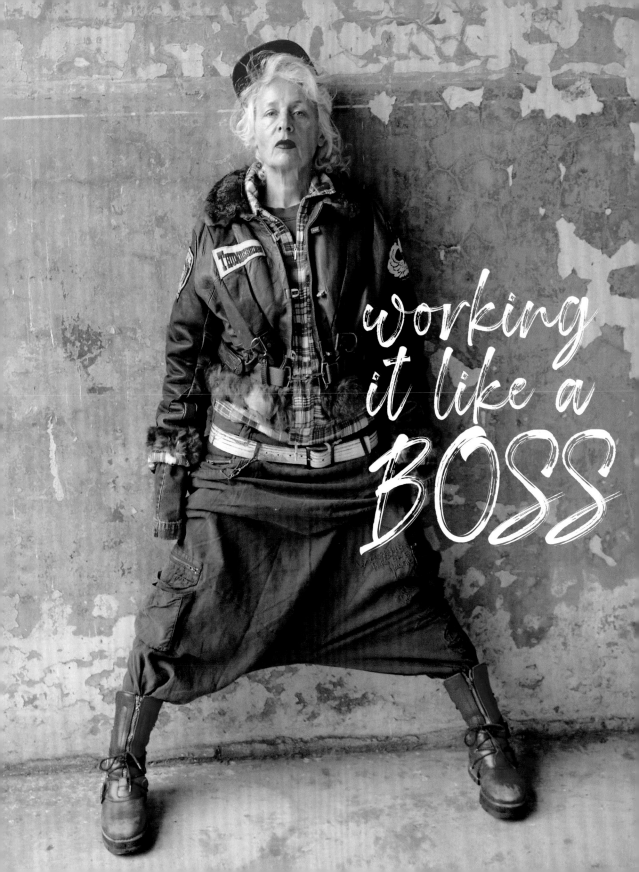

working
it like a
BOSS

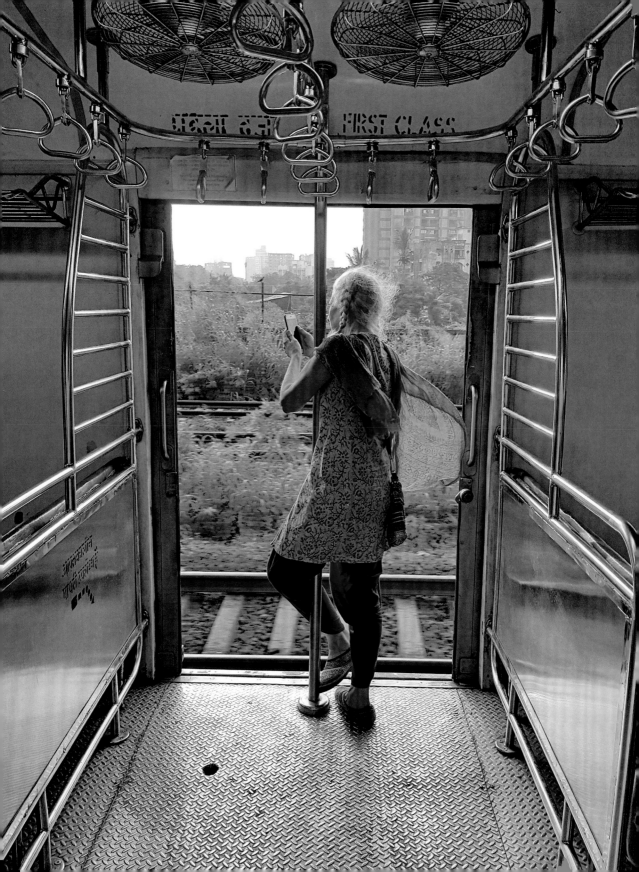

## WHISPERING TO THE WINDS, INSTAGRAM POST, MARCH 2017 (SHOWN ON PAGE 266)

This was shot in Jaipur in early 2017 and posted on my return to Australia, with the words: *"Whispering to the winds to take me there..."*

I frequently wear the same pieces for different functions, be they formal, informal, work or play. I am a multitasker and spontaneous, therefore my clothes must enable that lifestyle and those characteristics. I will wear the same pieces for travel, gardening, attending functions and doing my work; I don't change into a costume for different occasions.

My clothes reflect my mood, my attitude and how I feel I need to face the world each morning. I don't plan tomorrow's attire today; a mood can change overnight. Thankful to the wind that enabled this impromptu shot.

## LIVING THE DREAM, THE FIRST POST ON @MYWRINKLESAREMYSTRIPES, OCTOBER 2017

This non-event photo was taken by Big Man of me on a Mumbai train, captioned with the words *"Living the dream."*

The woman on the Saramai Jewels Instagram feed has become public property. I constantly battle with myself as to whether or not I should take it down. The numbers have grown exponentially as this woman becomes fodder for the grindstone of daily media, daily articles about older people on Instagram, people with grey hair, people with an 'inspiring' lifestyle. All these aspects are absolutely *not* how I self-identify.

## BACK TO IT, INSTAGRAM POST, NEWTOWN, MARCH 2018

This image was posted with the words:
*"Back to it*
*Comfort zone*
*Armoured up*
*Make of it what you will"*

My clothing has been my friend, my protector, my weapon and my armour. I dress to be invisible. What I wear has helped me live a fulfilling life, moving with ease across cultures, and subcultures, while reflecting my passage as a human who is now in her 60s and comfortable in her own skin.

The shock value of my dress means that people will look, then look away. I become invisible behind their confusion. It is a way for me to remain private.

Sometimes, my choice of clothing questions relationships between identities, plays with expectations, context and rules. By mixing components that emphasise the differentiations between subgroups, I challenge positions of power and vulnerability, weakness and strength, exclusion and membership.

I am my own tribe.

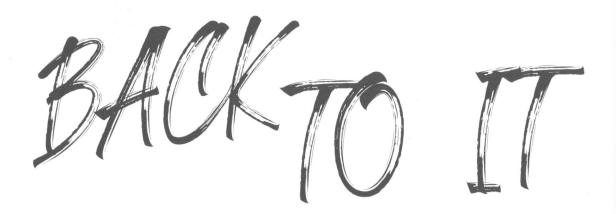

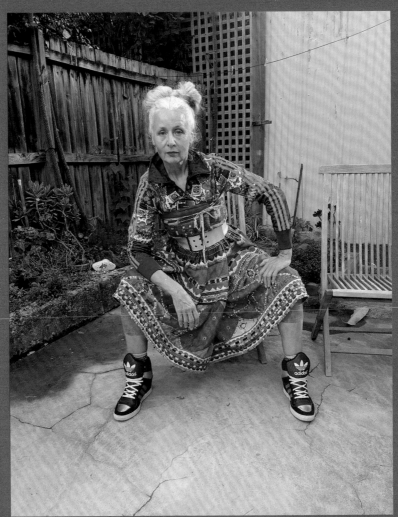

Back to it
Comfort zone
Armoured up
Make of it what you will

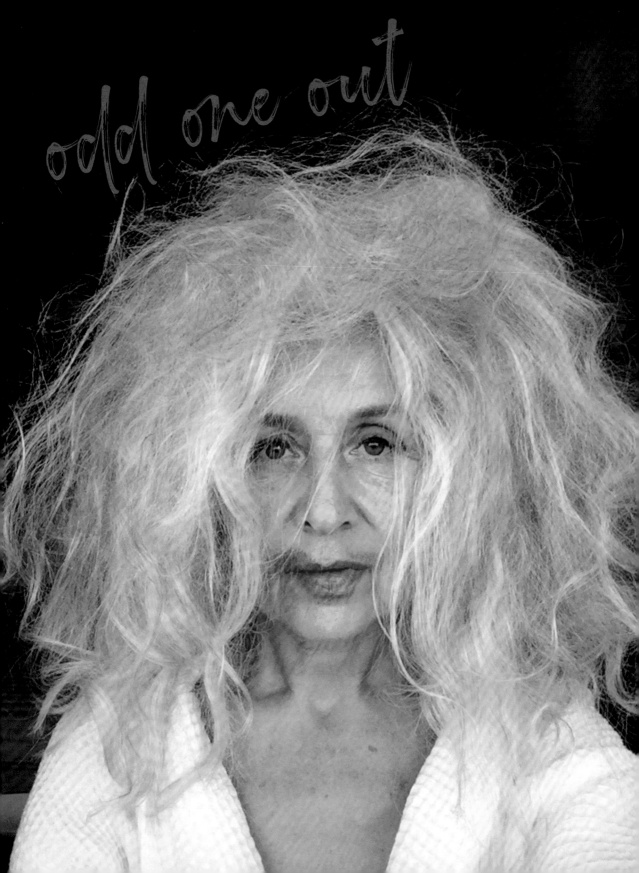

## ODD ONE OUT, INSTAGRAM POST, LONDON, JULY 2018

This image was posted with the words: *"It's OK to be the odd one out. Underneath we're all the same."*

This was a behind-the-scenes selfie, taken in the UK when I was one of the many people involved in an H&M 2018 'Holiday Season' campaign.

Since 2015, I have been lucky enough to have had the opportunity of working on a number of campaigns with a number of different genres of businesses and brands. This interesting experience has taken me to new places and given me a glimpse into another world – a world that is poles apart from my daily life. I have worked alongside models, hair-and-makeup artists and stylists – all incredibly talented people at the top of their game.

## HOME GIRL, INSTAGRAM POST, SYDNEY, AUGUST 2018 (SHOWN ON TITLE PAGE)

This image was posted with the words: *"Home girl."*

By my dress, I maintain my identity among a sea of high-street uniforms. In this instance, although the tracksuit is, indeed, a uniform, the wearer's attitude and age are the point of difference.

As a little girl, I resisted the ideal of 'looking nice', pleasing others and being pleasing to others. Being a tomboy meant that my choice of clothing had to be functional.

I have been like this for as long as I can remember.

*I have been like this for as long as I can remember.*

## COMING OR GOING, INSTAGRAM POST, LONDON, AUGUST 2018

Posted with the words: *"When you're not sure if you're coming or going."*

I am a modest, although challenging dresser. I do not dress to be sexually provocative; I seek to provoke thought and questions rather than attract. My concept of modesty is influenced by the places I have visited and the people I have met. My schooling meant that I never learnt how to deal with the gaze of men. Rarely do I expose more flesh than my lower legs and arms.

From my beloved India, I have learnt about the power of colour; the incredible combinations seen in nature and which are so readily and unabashedly transferred to garments, which, however tattered, are worn with love and pride.

I am interested in the relationship between frugality and excess, and how these conditions are not necessarily mutually exclusive. I am interested in discovering, too, how the use of oriental fabrics – silks, satins, prints, colours, surface decoration – however threadbare and worn they are, still touch on the exotic and otherworldly romanticism of a foreign land and different culture.

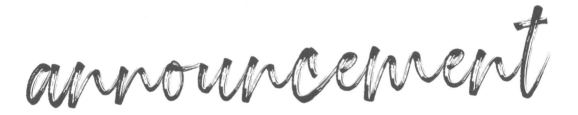

## THE ENTIRE COLLECTION HAS BEEN WITHDRAWN FROM SALE.

The author's children, Olivia and Natasha, are in negotiations regarding the placement of this Cabinet of Curiosities, their mother's personal collection, a 'Memento Hominem'.

These mundane, seemingly random, items from an ordinary life have, in fact, been curated with precision and are here seen through the prism of the personal as representations of events and memories. Remember only that you are human.

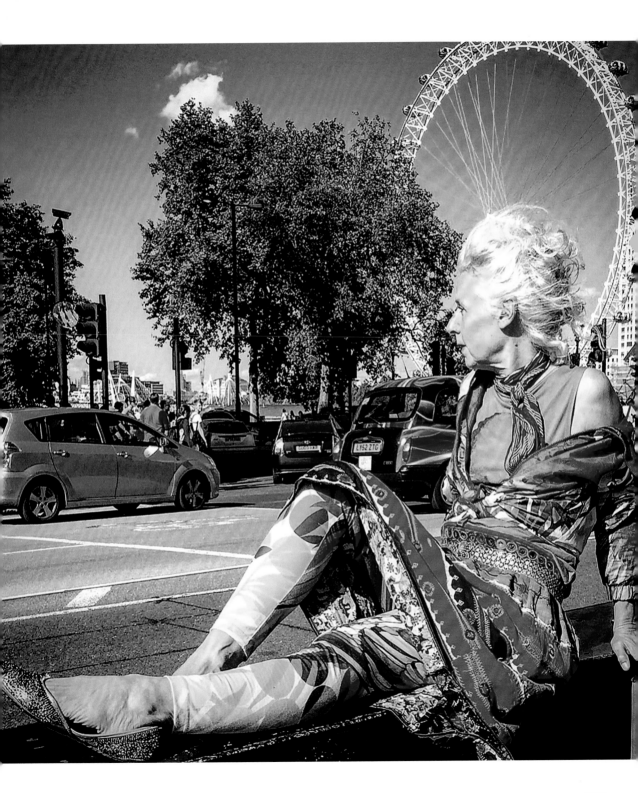

I know not from where I came and I know not where I'm going. I know not what the future holds. The older I become, the more I know that I know nothing.

I continue to learn to know myself.
Om Shanti. Shanti. Shanti.

# acknowledgements

Thanks to Kelly Doust for your persistence in making contact, your trust in, and understanding of, my compulsion to write an unusual kind of book; your love, patience and complete support throughout this entire roller-coaster of the amazing opportunity you have given me.

To my two guiding stars at Murdoch Books, major editing person Jane Price and major design person Megan Pigott, thank you for gently guiding me through this incredible experience.

Thanks to Sarah Odgers for your skilfully precise design work in placing the jigsaw pieces of images and words together, and to Sally Feldman for your wonderfully pedantic editing.

Thanks to Big Man for 'getting me'. Thanks for steadfastly being alongside me all the way, and specifically for working tirelessly with me on this project.

Thanks to my daughters, Olivia and Tash, for giving me space, love, strength and inspiration.

Thanks to my parents, Dorothy and Dickie Adams, and my twin sister, for giving me life.

Thanks to the Todywalla family, in particular Farokh, Yasmin and Jeroo, Kaizad and Monaz, Malcolm and Delna (and all the others, too many to mention by name!) for embracing me and my family completely into yours.

Thanks to Ari Seth Cohen for the way you have humbly changed the perception of ageing, and in so doing revolutionised the thinking of both the fashion and beauty industries. Thank you also for being a dear, dear friend, and for putting up with my crazy meltdowns when it all gets too much.

Thanks to Kirsten Albrecht and Marianne Davies for being my best girlfriends through good times and bad.

Thanks to Jason Parlett, my partner in op-shopping and story-swapping about all sorts of stuff.

Thanks to Jivamukti Sydney for keeping me sane.

Thanks to all those who have followed, liked, not liked, commented and shared on Insta. It is thanks to you that I have been given the opportunity to create this curious little book, about, basically, a load of old rubbish, seen through the prism of the personal.

And finally, a big thank-you to you, the reader; may you find your own Tessie Bear.

Published in 2020 by Murdoch Books, an imprint of Allen & Unwin

Murdoch Books Australia
83 Alexander Street, Crows Nest NSW 2065
Phone: +61 (0)2 8425 0100
murdochbooks.com.au
info@murdochbooks.com.au

Murdoch Books UK
Ormond House, 26–27 Boswell Street,
London, WC1N 3JZ
Phone: +44 (0) 20 8785 5995
murdochbooks.co.uk
info@murdochbooks.co.uk

For corporate orders & custom publishing contact our business
development team at salesenquiries@murdochbooks.com.au

Publisher: Kelly Doust
Editorial Manager: Jane Price
Creative Manager and Cover Designer: Megan Pigott
Designer: Sarah Odgers
Editor: Sally Feldman
Production Director: Lou Playfair

ISBN 978 1 76052 495 1 Australia
ISBN 978 1 91163 244 3 UK

A catalogue record for this
book is available from the
National Library of Australia

A catalogue record for this book is available from the British Library
Colour reproduction by Splitting Image Colour Studio Pty Ltd, Clayton, Victoria
Printed by C & C Offset Printing Co Ltd, China

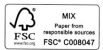
The paper in this book is FSC® certified.
FSC® promotes environmentally responsible,
socially beneficial and economically viable
management of the world's forests.

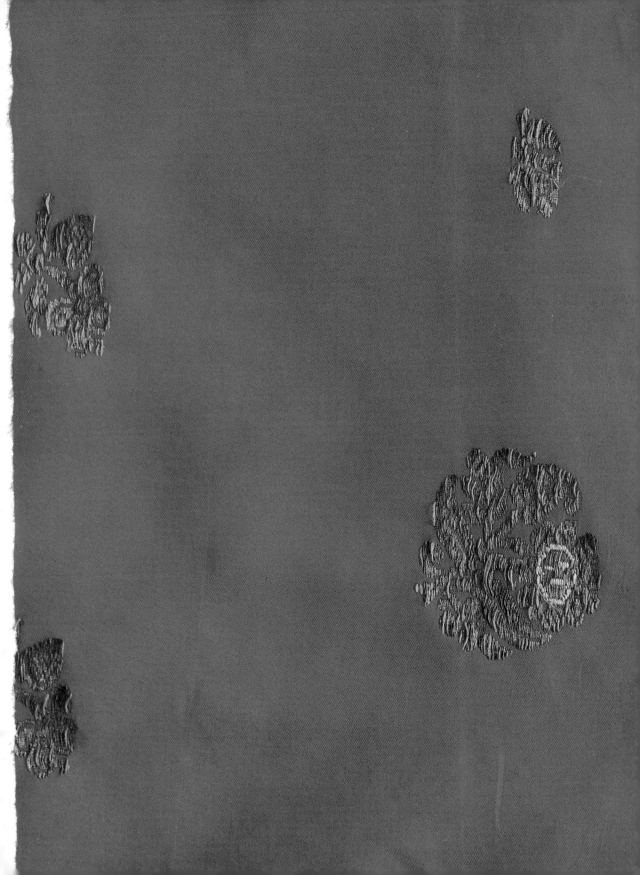

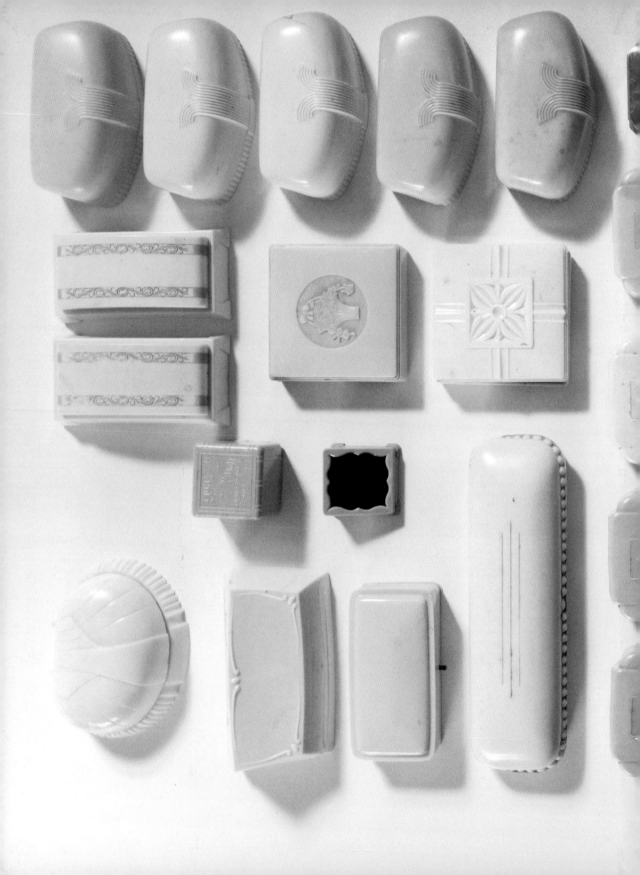